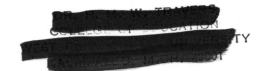
D1616911

Skilled Performance:

PERCEPTUAL AND MOTOR SKILLS

Skilled Performance;
PERCEPTUAL AND MOTOR SKILLS

A. T. Welford
UNIVERSITY OF ADELAIDE

Lyle E. Bourne, Jr.   Consulting Editor
University of Colorado at Boulder

Scott, Foresman and Company

Glenview, Illinois
Dallas, Tex.   Oakland, N.J.   Palo Alto, Cal.   Tucker, Ga.   Brighton, England

Library of Congress Cataloging in Publication Data

Welford, Alan Traviss. Skilled Performance: Perceptual and Motor Skills.

Bibliography: p. 169. Includes index.
1. Perceptual-motor learning.   2. Intellect.
3. Social interaction.
I. Title.   [DNLM: 1. Motor skills.
2. Social perception.   3. Social behavior.
4. Intelligence.   5. Perception.   BF431. W445]
BF295. W43   152.3   75-35537   ISBN 0-673-07709-8
1 2 3 4 5-RRC-80 79 78 75

ACKNOWLEDGMENTS FOR FIGURES AND TABLES

FIGURES

(2.6) Sherif, M., and Hovland, C. *Social Judgment.* New Haven: Yale University Press, 1961, p. 53. Reprinted by permission. (2.9) Vickers, D. "A cyclic mode of perceptual alternation." *Perception,* 1972, *1,* 31–38. Reprinted by permission.

(3.1) Adapted from Bricker, P. D. "The identification of redundant stimulus patterns." *Journal of Experimental Psychology, 49,* 73–81. Copyright © 1955 by the American Psychological Association. Reprinted by permission. (3.2) Adapted from Hochberg, J., and McAlister, E. "A quantitative approach to figural 'goodness.'" *Journal of Experimental Psychology, 46,* 361–64. Copyright © 1953 by the American Psychological Association. Reprinted by permission. (3.4; 3.5) Vickers, D. From A. T. Welford, *Fundamentals of Skill.* London: Methuen & Co., Ltd., 1968. Reprinted by permission.

(4.1) Based on data from Hick, W. E. "On the rate of gain of information." *Quarterly Journal of Experimental Psychology,* 1952, *4,* 11–26. Reprinted by permission. (4.2) Crossman, E. R. F. W. "Entropy and choice time: The effect of frequency unbalance on choice response." *Quarterly Journal of Experimental Psychology,* 1953, *5,* 41–51. Reprinted by permission.

(5.1) Based on data from Vince, M. A. "Corrective movements in a pursuit task." *Quarterly Journal of Experimental Psychology,* 1948, *1,* 85–103. Reprinted by permission. (5.2; 5.3) Welford, A. T., Norris, A. H., & Shock, N. M. "Speed and accuracy of movement and their changes with age." *Acta Psychologica,* 1969, *30,* 3–15. Reprinted by permission of the North-Holland Publishing Company, Amsterdam. (5.4) From Welford, A. T. "Single-channel operation in the brain." *Acta Psychologica,* 1967, *27,* 5–22. Based on data from Conrad, R. "Speed and load stress in sensorimotor skill." *British Journal of Industrial Medicine,* 1951, *8,* 1–7. Reprinted by permission.

(6.1) Wright, J. M. von. *An Experimental Study of Human Serial Learning.* Societas Scientiarum Fennica. Commentationes Humanarum Litterarum, 1957, *23,* No. 1. (6.2) Wright, J. M. von. "A note on the role of 'guidance' in learning." *British Journal of Psychology,* 1957, *48,* 133–37. Reprinted by permission of the Cambridge University Press. (6.3) Based on data from Wallace, J. G. "Some studies of perception in relation to age." *British Journal of Psychology,* 1956, *47,* 283–297. Reprinted by permission of the Cambridge University Press. (6.4) Crossman, E. R. F. W. "A theory of the acquisition of speed-skill." *Ergonomics,* 1959, *2,* 153–66. Reprinted by permission.

TABLES

(4.3) Adapted from data in Brainard, R. W., Irby, T. S., Fitts, P. M., & Alluisi, E. A. "Some variables influencing the rate of gain of information." *Journal of Experimental Psychology, 63,* 105–10. Copyright © 1962 by the American Psychological Association. Reprinted by permission.

(6.1) Szafran, J., & Welford, A. T. "On the relation between transfer and difficulty of initial task." *Quarterly Journal of Experimental Psychology,* 1950, *2,* 88–94. Reprinted by permission.

Table of contents

Foreword

The contemporary field of skilled human performance owes its beginning largely to a small group of researchers working in Great Britain during the late '40s, '50s, and '60s, prominent among them K. J. W. Craik, W. E. Hick, A. T. Welford, and D. E. Broadbent. Their studies focused on the development of an information-communication theory of human behavior. Fitts and others in the United States had similar ideas and the two movements, implemented in computer modeling, merged together and evolved into what today we call the information processing approach to psychology. In the present volume, Professor A. T. Welford gives a contemporary account of how these ideas can be used to organize and to interpret the facts of human performance.

This book is a masterpiece of logic and organization. Each paragraph, page, and chapter flows from its predecessor. Professor Welford takes as his main theme the idea that skill can be defined as the effective use of one's capacities which are, of course, subject to change through experience and practice. Skills are the products of learning. They constitute at any particular time the sum total of a given individual's "know-how." The coverage of the book is broader than its name, Skilled Performance: Perceptual and Motor Skills, might imply. The breadth of his coverage is exemplified in the manner in which Professor Welford takes the basic facts of perceptual and motor skill, derived largely from the psychological laboratory, and extends them to an interpretation of decision, cognitive, and even social psychological processes. The development is one which students are likely to appreciate, for it shows in a compelling way the manner in which *psychological research can make sense of contemporary problems which touch all of our lives.*

The book is a pleasure to read. There is a minimum of jargon and a maximum of plain, straightforward talk. The emphasis is on basic psychological processes, but there are plenty of applications to show the importance of this work for those who might not be deeply dedicated to research. This book will be important not only as a textbook for courses in learning and human performance but also as a source of new ideas for research in these areas. It has been my pleasure to serve as academic editor for this volume. Professor Welford's skill and experience both in his subject matter and in the art of clear writing have made my job a simple and pleasurable one.

LYLE E. BOURNE, JR.
Consulting Editor

Preface

This book is about skills: motor, perceptual, intellectual, and social skills. Its purpose is to indicate what appear to be the principles and concepts common to all these areas.

The essential thesis of the book is that skills lie in the efficient and effective use of capacities as the result of experience and practice. Different types of capacity are surveyed in turn, in each case by looking first at their main principles of operation and then examining the extent to which their use is improved with practice or training. The capacities concerned relate not only to motor activities but to the whole range of cognitive and decisional processes.

The aim is to sketch the main outlines of the studies that have come to be known as "skills research," picking out what appear, on present knowledge, to be salient points and fitting them into a broad overall pattern. To achieve this, treatment has had to be highly selective, often focusing primarily on one view of a problem and leaving it to the reader to pursue others by way of references. Also, the amount of evidence available varies greatly from one area to another, so that some topics are covered in detail while others have had to be sketched more lightly, pointing to substantial areas of ignorance as well as of knowledge. It is my hope, however, that this approach will serve to give a fuller perspective to the potential as well as the actual study of human skills.

The treatment throughout is in fundamental, theoretical terms. The last thirty or so years have clearly shown, however, that interest in concepts of skill and proof of their validity come from their application to practical problems of industry, the armed services, sport, music, and education. Theoretical points have therefore been illustrated with examples from real life and attention drawn to potential applications in these various fields.

I am grateful to Dr. N. H. Kirby, Dr. T. J. Nettelbeck, and Mr. G. A. Smith for permission to use unpublished data, and to these and also to Dr. J. M. T. Brebner, Professor I. D. John, and Dr. D. Vickers for helpful suggestions and comments. My thanks are due to Mrs. M. L. Blaber and Mrs. H. M. Holmes for tackling the difficult task of translating my manuscript into typescript, and to Mrs. J. D. Hallett and Mrs. H. Lomax for their work on the diagrams.

I must also thank the Publishers' editorial staff for the careful and detailed way in which they have edited the typescript. Their work in bringing my text more into line with familiar textbook idiom has undoubtedly made it easier for many readers. The resulting style is, however, not always mine.

A. T. WELFORD
Adelaide
South Australia

Skilled Performance:
PERCEPTUAL AND MOTOR SKILLS

What is skill?

1

Until the 1940s, the study of skill was largely confined to industry. People were regarded as skilled when they were able to carry out a trade or activity that involved knowledge, judgment, accuracy, and manual dexterity, qualifications usually acquired as the result of long training. In contrast, an unskilled worker was not expected to do anything which could not be learned in a relatively short time. Semiskilled jobs were considered to involve some of the characteristics of skilled work but to demand a less extensive training period, generally lasting weeks or months rather than years. This industrial definition of skill, expressed fundamentally in terms of the amount of training and experience required for effective performance, has remained essentially the same to the present time.

However, technological developments in World War II brought about a broader interest in the concept of skill. The development of weapons, high-speed aircraft, radar, and many other devices reached such a point that the interaction of man and machine was no longer limited primarily by the machine but by the human operator. No matter how rigorously operators were selected and how thoroughly trained, they were unable to control the machines they had to work with satisfactorily or to realize the potentialities of them fully.

Thus it became imperative to develop a better understanding of the many facets of human performance and of how these facets might be matched with machines. While this could be done to some extent by training the operators, it was mainly achieved by taking human capacities and limitations into account in the design of the machines. The insights gained from research with military equipment have, in turn, expanded the interest of industry from its almost exclusive concern with manual operations to include process control and office work, as well as attempts to understand the human factors involved in managerial decision making.

More recently, the scope of research on skills has been extended by increasingly sophisticated studies of performance in games and athletic activities. The reasons for this development are not entirely clear, but seem to have been fostered by two trends. First, interest has been aroused in the competitive standards of several sports that have become highly popular and lucrative entertainments. Second, there is a widespread belief that exercise protects against heart disease and many other ills of middle age.

In all these research areas, skill is thought of as a quality of performance which does not depend solely upon a person's fundamental, innate capacities, but must be developed through training, practice, and experience. Skill essentially depends upon learning, but to say that skill is merely a facet of learning would be misleading; it also includes the concepts of efficiency and economy in performance. Development of skill goes far beyond the registration of items, or associations between items, normally studied under the heading of learning. Modern concepts of skill stress the flexibility with which a skilled operator reaches a given end on different occasions, varying specific actions according to precise circumstances. Thus, all action is the result of a complex computation based on data from many sources—not only from the eyes and ears, but from posture, environmental sources, and the results of past actions and future aims. Unlike traditional learning studies, investigations of skill speak not of responses to stimuli but of "strategies" and "procedures"—larger organizations which, although less precisely defined, are closer to describing the units of performance that seem to occur in normal, everyday life. To put it another way, although basic human capacities are not sufficient to produce skills, they form the necessary basis of their development; skills represent particular ways of using capacities in relation to environmental demands, with human being and external situation together forming a functional "system."

To understand skill we must study human capacities and the mechanisms underlying them, in order to see how they can be used more effectively and efficiently to manipulate the world and meet its demands. In this chapter, we shall outline the main functional mechanisms within the organism which make up the chain leading from sensory input to motor action and which must underlie skilled performance. In later chapters we shall look at each of these mechanisms in turn, considering its potentialities and limitations, and the extent to which its functioning can be improved in the course of experience.

The chain of mechanisms

The diagram in Figure 1.1 summarizes the results of a great many researches into human performance which have been designed to identify the principal

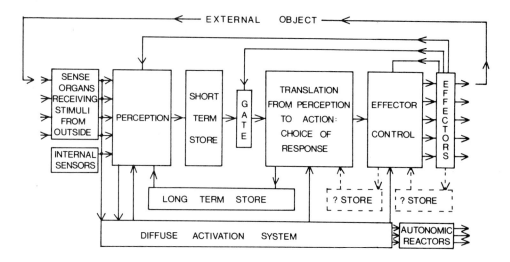

Figure 1.1. *Hypothetical block diagram of the human sensory-motor system.*

mechanisms involved in skill and how they interact. It must be emphasized that the diagram is not intended to portray anatomical features of the organism. While some of the "boxes," such as those for the sense organs and effectors, represent identifiable bodily structures, the main central stages denote what appear to be distinct *functions*, not at present clearly assigned to particular brain structures. We shall take this diagram as our starting point, looking briefly at its several parts prior to their fuller treatment in subsequent chapters.

The peripheral stages

The sense organs, shown at the extreme left of the diagram, fall into two groups. One group consists of receptors which receive data from external sources—eyes, ears, nose, mouth, and skin. The other group may be divided into two categories. First, there are internal receptors in muscles, tendons, and joints which supply data which seldom impinge on consciousness but play an important part in the control of movement. Second, there are a number of less understood sensors which measure the state of blood chemistry, of dehydration, and of other bodily conditions, and which seem to act directly on the brain.

The effectors, shown at the extreme right of the diagram, also fall into two groups, one including the hands, feet, vocal organs, and the other instruments of the voluntary muscles; the other consisting of the various reactors of the autonomic system, which are not normally under voluntary control.

The main central divisions

The three major divisions of the central mechanisms deal respectively with perception, translating perception to action, and the controlling of action.

If, for example, a tiger were to walk into the room, it would be one thing to recognize what it was, quite another to decide what to do about it, and still another to carry out any action required. Viewed in more detail, the process starts with data from the various sense organs feeding into the perceptual mechanism. There they are coordinated and supplemented by data from the long-term memory store until a point is reached when they are ready to form the basis of action. They are then fed through into the translation mechanism, either immediately or after a delay in the short-term store. The translation mechanism computes a response, the orders for which are passed on to the central effector mechanism, which programs a phased sequence of muscular action to execute the response.

The means of identifying such stages and what is done in each have been discussed in detail by Sternberg (1969b). For our present purpose it is sufficient to note that the separation between perception of signal and choice of response is indicated by experiments on reaction time in which the directness with which a signal was linked to a response was varied, thus varying the amount of "work" required by the translation mechanism once the signal had been identified. As we shall see in Chapter 4, reaction time rises in a highly predictable way with the number of possible signals that may occur on any occasion, and the number of possible corresponding responses. The rate of increase is, however, much less when signals are closely related to corresponding responses. For example, when responses have to be made by pressing keys under different fingers, the rate of increase in reaction time is less when the signals are vibrations delivered to the tips of the fingers concerned, than when they are lights on a panel (Leonard, 1959; Smith, 1976). It is also less when lights are immediately next to their corresponding keys, than when they are scattered in a random pattern on a panel (Crossman, 1956). The rise is also less when, although several different signals are given, a response is required to only one, than when different responses are required to two or more (Donders, 1868; Brebner & Gordon, 1962, 1964; see also Welford, 1968).

Further support for separating perception from choice of response, and indications that the choice of response should also be separated from the phasing and execution of action, comes from experiments on reaction time which followed an important theoretical paper by Craik (1948). During the 1940s several studies had been made of performance at tracking tasks. These studies involved moving a lever, or turning a steering wheel, in order to keep a pointer in line with a target which moved irregularly from side to side. Interest in this task originated with attempts to improve the aiming of weapons by the crews of warships and tanks, but it has continued because of its theoretical significance and obvious similarity to the steering of vehicles.

Craik noticed that the pointer did not follow the target smoothly, but showed a series of oscillations, implying that correction of misalignment between pointer and target was not made continuously, but at discrete intervals of about half a second. Searching for a reason, he was led to ask why an appreciable reaction time elapsed between the presentation of a signal and the emergence of a response to it. He argued that if reaction time was due to the signal having to be transmitted down a long chain of synapses to activate the response, as in a "telephone exchange" theory of brain operation, there was no reason why a continuous signal should not lead to a continuous response, even if a little late. He suggested as an alternative that the signal started a computation in the brain, and that while this computation was going on, further input which might disturb it was blocked. Following this view, the intake of data and the initiation of responses would be intermittent—the results of a series of discrete computations.

Craik suggested that this view could be tested by presenting signals for action at varying intervals, to see if subjects responded more slowly to signals coming at very short intervals after other signals than when the intervals between signals were longer. The many experiments subsequently carried out have been summarized by several authors (e.g., Bertelson, 1966; Welford, 1967, 1968; Herman & Kantowitz, 1970; Posner & Klein, 1973). A typical example consists of giving the subject a light signal to respond to as quickly as possible by pressing a key. During the reaction time to the signal—that is, between the time at which the light appears and the key is pressed—a second light must be responded to by pressing a second key. The result is that reaction time to the second signal is longer than if the interval between the two had been greater.

Interpretation of such experiments has not always been easy and has led to a good deal of controversy. However, the extent of the delay is such as to suggest that the central processes, or some part of them, cannot begin to deal with the second signal until they have finished dealing with the first and the response to it has been initiated. The data from the second signal thus have to be stored for a fraction of a second until the central mechanisms are free. Close analysis of the evidence suggests that the operation can be broadly represented as in Figure 1.2 (Welford, 1968). From this it can be seen that the delay is due to the translation mechanism dealing with only one signal at a time. It is assumed that as soon as the first signal has been passed to the translation mechanism the gate shown in Figure 1.1 closes, protecting the computation in the translation mechanism from interference by further input until the gate is opened again. The opening of the gate and the beginning of a new calculation by the translation mechanism seems to depend on feedback from the initiation of response to the first signal. Indications that this is so come from a somewhat different line of research in which feedback from the response is delayed. The subject is asked to write a word on paper with the writing hand hidden from direct view. The hand can be seen, however, on a television screen with a running delay of half a second or so. Under such conditions writing is slow and hesitant and letters tend to be repeated, as if the orders for their execution had not been cancelled and replaced by those for the next action (Smith, 1962; Smith & Smith, 1962).

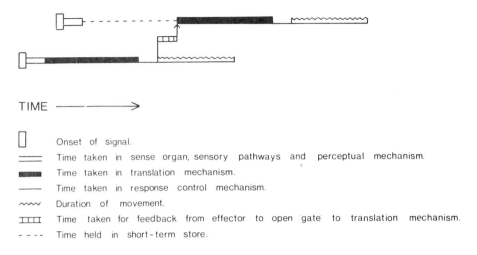

TIME ———————⟶

⎕   Onset of signal.

═══   Time taken in sense organ, sensory pathways and perceptual mechanism.

▄▄▄▄   Time taken in translation mechanism.

———   Time taken in response control mechanism.

⌒⌒⌒   Duration of movement.

ⅢⅢ   Time taken for feedback from effector to open 'gate' to translation mechanism.

- - - -   Time held in short-term store.

Figure 1.2. *Diagram of the single-channel hypothesis for cases in which a signal for action arrives during the reaction time to a previous signal.*

It should be noted in passing, that if the second signal comes within about 80–100 milliseconds (msec) of the first, the pattern of responding shown in Figure 1.2 is commonly replaced by one in which the reaction time to the first signal is longer than normal, and both signals are responded to simultaneously in a coordinated, double response. In other words, it looks as if the gate takes an appreciable time to close, during which the second signal can be passed to the translation mechanism along with the first, so that both are dealt with together.

Figure 1.2 shows that the second signal can be perceived while the translation mechanism is selecting the response to the first, and that the translation mechanism can be selecting a response to the second signal while the response to the first is being executed. Thus in tracking, the observation of each misalignment between target and follower and the decision about the correction needed can be carried out while the preceding correction is being made. The overlapping of these operations is also shown in a number of everyday tasks. For example, a close analysis of the performance of typists makes it clear that they perceive and process data from copy and type it out in groups of several letters or words, and that as they type one group, they are taking in the next (Shaffer, 1973). The same seems to be true in the playing of a musical instrument; the score is read and notes are played not singly but in whole phrases, and while one phrase is being played the next one is being read. The size of the group dealt with in such tasks appears to increase with practice, and was regarded by Bryan & Harter (1897, 1899), in their classical studies of Morse code operators, as a measure of skill.

The way of conceiving the operation of the central mechanisms set out in Figure 1.2 has come to be known as the *single-channel hypothesis*.

It is clear that the single channel lies in the translation mechanism which deals with only one signal, or group of signals, at a time. This hypothesis is of fundamental importance in explaining the limitations of many kinds of continuous performance, which will be discussed in Chapter 5.

The memory stores

Of the two memory stores shown in Figure 1.1, the short-term one is a buffer store which holds limited amounts of data for brief periods, after which they are completely forgotten. The holding mechanism is commonly assumed to be some kind of brain activity depending on self-regenerating circuits of neurons, analogous to the dynamic memory of some early electronic computers (Hebb, 1949). Data in the long-term store must be held in some more enduring form, either a biochemical or a submicroscopic structural change in brain cells, which can survive severe insults to the brain and also conditions such as near freezing during which brain activity is at a standstill (Andjus et al., 1956). The long-term store holds data for long periods—up to several years at least—and it is sometimes claimed that nothing registered in it is ever completely forgotten. Whether or not this is so, it is certainly true that vast amounts of data are stored there during an individual's lifetime.

Normally, the two stores work closely together, so that their contributions are often difficult to separate. In fact, some researchers have claimed that the memory stores should not be distinguished. However, evidence of their separateness comes from clinical studies which show that one store may be severely impaired while the other is little affected (e.g., Symonds, 1966; Wickelgren, 1968). Further evidence is provided by Baddeley (1966a, b), who showed that the two systems produced different types of error: in short-term memory confusions tend to occur between words which are acoustically similar, while in long-term memory confusions tend to take place between words which are similar in meaning.

Additional indications that there are two stores come from studies of the retrograde amnesia which follows temporary loss of consciousness from a blow on the head, or from other violent assault on the brain such as electroconvulsive shock (for a review see Glickman, 1961). Upon regaining consciousness, the individual may be unable to remember anything that happened during a substantial period prior to the event, except perhaps in a fragmentary and disordered manner. Gradually the memories return, usually the more distant first. There remains, however, a short period of a few seconds or minutes the memories of which are permanently lost. We can envisage that the more distant memories, held in the long-term store, are not recoverable during the period of amnesia because the assault has produced random activity in the brain which blurs the pattern of its action. The few seconds or minutes permanently lost represent data held in the short-term store which had not yet been passed to the long-term store.

There has been some controversy as to whether the short-term store is located before or after the perceptual stage shown in Figure 1.1. Several experiments in which a substantial amount of material has been flashed on a screen at one time have shown that, although subjects cannot repoduce all the material, they can nevertheless reproduce any one part of it indicated to them within half a second or so after the presentation. This implies that the whole of the material has been briefly stored somewhere peripheral to the perceptual mechanism in which it is identified (e.g., Sperling, 1960; Averbach & Sperling, 1961). However, this "iconic" visual storage is far too ephemeral to account for short-term retention over a period of several seconds.

What at first sight also appeared to be evidence for a peripheral store came from experiments by Broadbent (1954, 1957) who presented pairs of digits simultaneously, one to each ear, and found a marked tendency for subjects to recall all the digits from one ear before recalling any digits heard by the other. Thus digits presented

Right ear	7	2	5
Left ear	1	8	3

tended to be recalled 7 2 5 1 8 3 rather than 7 1 2 8 5 3. This suggested that there were two stores, one pertaining to each ear, which were visited in turn. However, other similar experiments (e.g., Gray & Wedderburn, 1960) in which different classes of material were presented, have found recall to be class by class rather than ear by ear, thus

Right ear	CYC-	7	STYLE
Left ear	1	LO-	3

tended to be recalled CYCLOSTYLE 173. This style of recall is obviously based on data which have been combined from the two ears and interpreted before being stored. It therefore implies that storage has taken place after rather than before perceptual processing and identification.

The location of the long-term store is also open to question. The choice appears to be between the placement shown in Figure 1.1 and incorporation into the main central mechanisms, especially the perceptual mechanism. Much of the evidence can be accounted for with either arrangement. Bartlett (1932) showed that material in the long-term store is not the actual data presented to a subject but is the subject's reactions to it, and it has been repeatedly shown that active response to material, rather than passive observation, makes for quicker and more thorough learning. For example, Gates (1917) showed that rote learning of words and syllables was more thorough if reading of the material was alternated with attempts to recite it, rather than with reading alone. It can be argued that since there is always some tendency to recite material as it is read, even if only silently, nothing would be learned unless some response was made. At first such response was thought to be effective because of the actual actions involved, but later studies by von Wright (1957b) and by Belbin (1958, 1964; Belbin & Downs, 1964) have shown that it depends on the subject making active choices instead of passively observing. We shall discuss this work further in Chapter 6.

These effects of active response suggest a long-term store fed from the translation mechanism as shown in Figure 1.1, but they would also be consistent with storage in the perceptual, or perhaps the translation, mechanism if it could be argued that active response requires the development of more fully differentiated states in these mechanisms, and thus of more sharply defined traces than does mere observation of data. Indications in favor of the scheme diagrammed in Figure 1.1, however, come from the everyday observation that if we do not immediately recognize an object, we seem to search around in memory for a match to it. In other words, we perceive the object clearly and then try first one and then another area of stored memory in order to categorize it.

It looks, in fact, as if items or sets of items are in turn read into the perceptual mechanism from the long-term store until a match is obtained. A further indication comes from the fact that if a string of, say, 10 digits, letters, or disconnected words is read to a subject who is asked to repeat them immediately, the items presented early show signs of having been recovered from the long-term store. Presumably the short-term store has insufficient capacity to contain the whole string, and the earlier items are put through into the long-term store if they are retained at all. Several of these earlier items are retained even if the later items are recalled first, implying that they have somehow been shunted for storage off the main line of information flow.

Perhaps the truth is that both types of long-term storage exist. Patients with brain damage, whose long-term memory has been lost, are still able to recognize and react to everyday objects around them, which implies that there is still some structuring of perception and action by experience. Brain damaged individuals have, however, lost the wealth of detailed recognition that must obviously reside in long-term storage. Such detail should still be available if the stores were in the perceptual or translation mechanisms, but would be unavailable if the link from a separate long-term store to the perceptual mechanism shown in Figure 1.1 has been broken.

These same patients, although unable either to learn or to recall cognitive details, may still retain and even acquire motor skills (Corkin, 1968; Milner, 1970). This seems to imply some storage in, or associated with, the translation and central effector mechanisms independent of that associated with the perceptual mechanism. Little is understood about such storage, and its tentative indication in Figure 1.1 by dotted lines is little more than a guess.

Feedback
Performance hardly ever consists of only one run through the chain of mechanisms from sense organs to effectors. Even relatively simple actions,

such as picking up a glass or opening a door, involve an iterative process in which an initial action, such as making a reaching movement, is followed by further smaller movements, each of which depends for its precise form on the outcome of one before. In other words, data from the effector action and its results on the external world are fed back as part of the sensory input for the next run through the chain, as indicated by the main feedback loop shown at the top of Figure 1.1.

The most obvious and important effect of such feedback is the correction of error. For example, a blindfolded subject who tries to draw a series of lines each of a given length—say, 12 cms—will probably make substantial errors. If, however, the subject is shown or told after each attempt how the line just drawn compares with 12 cms, accuracy will quickly improve. If, in further trials, such "knowledge of results" is withdrawn, performance at once deteriorates (Thorndike, 1931; Macpherson et al., 1948). Dees and Grindley (1951) found the immediate deterioration of performance was due to the tendency of subjects to overshoot the specified target—a finding which implies that the feedback provided by the knowledge of results held a potentially over-responsive mechanism in check.

What appears to happen is that some standard is set up in the perceptual mechanism, the feedback from each response is compared with this, and the "orders" passed to the translation mechanism, and by it in turn to the effector mechanism, are modified according to whether the results of the last response were too great or too small. Performance over a series of trials is thus once again seen to be *flexible* in the sense that there is a steady overall aim, with detailed performance differing at each attempt to reach it. The principle is important, and applies to many types of performance, especially those involving crafts, trades, or sports where expertness requires a high degree of skill. We should stress again that none of these performances can be satisfactorily conceived in terms of particular stimuli leading to particular responses in the way postulated by classical stimulus-response theories. Instead, each action is individually computed according to the detailed circumstances of the moment and the results of previous action.

This same principle underlies the modern approach to motivation: a discrepancy between the present situation and some optimum is detected and action is set in motion which continues until the discrepancy is eliminated. We may note in passing that feedback, in addition to its corrective function, seems to have a motivational effect in that successful manipulation of the external world appears to produce both satisfaction and a tendency to continue or repeat the activity concerned (Gibbs & Brown, 1956).

Of the other feedback loops shown in Figure 1.1, the loop from the effector end to the gate guarding the translation mechanism has already been mentioned. The loop from the effectors to their central control mechanism is one of many which have been demonstrated by neurological studies, and is important in the detailed muscular control required to produce smooth action. This is shown by the extreme clumsiness of people in whom the loop has been impaired by neurological injury, or by disease such as *tabes dorsalis* (Gibbs, 1954), or artificially blocked (Laszlo, 1966).

The diffuse activation system

Incoming data from the sense organs build up detailed activation in the main chain of central mechanisms which leads to specific action. Neurological evidence has also shown that there is a secondary system which supplies a more diffuse stimulation and causes a widespread nonspecific activation. This secondary system appears to be the basis of *arousal,* not only making the difference between sleep and wakefulness, but also providing subtle changes in the level of arousal from moment to moment. For example, in a person driving a car, the level of arousal appears to be raised briefly by any incident, however trivial, such as passing or being passed or crossing an intersection (Hulbert, 1957; Michaels, 1960; Taylor, 1964).

The activation mechanism, which is centered in the brain stem, sends diffuse impulses to the cortex which increase its sensitivity and responsiveness. The center receives inputs from the various sensory channels so that it responds to any stimulation. It also seems to have connections from the perceptual mechanism so that it reacts to any situation which requires effort or threatens departure from optimum conditions. It is thus the mediator of certain generalized reactions to stress and motivation. Subjectively, the activation mechanism is associated with emotions and feelings. It appears to have connections with all the main central stages, enhancing their activity at times of high demand and reducing activity under monotonous conditions. It also has connections with the autonomic nervous system, whose activities are commonly used as indices of arousal.

The arousal system appears to be distinct from the main central stages. This impression gains support from experimental results which have shown that a signal to speed up a movement can become effective without incurring the delay that would normally follow from the closing of the gate between the perceptual and translation mechanisms (Vince & Welford, 1967). Megaw (1972a, b, 1974) has shown that a signal to extend or reverse a movement may also appear to get past the gate. Its effect, however, is not to alter the precise times at which the various muscles contract, but to produce more intense contraction by all the muscles concerned, so that they become effective a little sooner than they otherwise would. In short, the signal which bypasses the gate does not require any fresh calculation by the translation mechanism, but merely an intensification of action already decided.

Signals for intensification seem to be more effective in bypassing the gate than are those for diminution or cessation of activity, presumably because the latter tend to call for an active opposition to the program of muscular contractions already decided, and thus for a fresh calculation by the translation mechanism. The author once put this point to a skilled tennis player who remarked that it was in line with instruction in many sports—a stroke should always begin slowly as it is easier to speed up than to slow down.

Types of skill

Looking at the system as a whole, the human sensory-motor chain and the external situation in which it operates can be seen to form a *servo system*. Performance depends on the characteristics of the two parts of the system taken together, so that if performance is to be understood, both human capacities and the demands of the environment must be specified and measured *in the same terms*. Doing so has opened up important new approaches to many situations in which people work with machines, leading on the theoretical side to the study of *cybernetics*, and on the practical side to *ergonomics* or *human engineering*. It is clear also that similar principles can be applied to social interaction, in that any two or more people in communication with one another must inevitably form a feedback system, each receiving input from others, processing it, and using it to shape action which the others observe (Welford, 1966a, b, 1968).

The operation of each of the three main central mechanisms in Figure 1.1 seems capable of showing skill. What is commonly recognized as *perceptual skill* consists essentially in the coding of, and giving coherence to, the multitudinous sensory data that pour in through the sense organs, and in linking these data to material stored in memory to give them context in both space and time. Individuals obviously differ in their levels of skill in this respect. Some people perceive objects and recognize their meaning more readily and fully than others do; these differences appear to be at least partly due to experience which has made certain codings familiar and led to expectations associated with particular stimulus patterns. Perceptual skill thus seems to be bound up with close interaction between the perceptual mechanism and the long-term memory store.

At the other end of the chain are *motor skills* such as riding a bicycle, making golf or tennis strokes, or playing a musical instrument. In all these activities certain well practiced motor coordinations become seemingly automatic, being carried on without detailed conscious attention. Because of this, it is tempting to assume that they reside solely in the central effector stage. However, almost all motor skills depend upon a close interplay between action and sensory input, and thus appear to involve the other central mechanisms as well.

Many, perhaps the majority, of the most important skills in real life are concerned with the translation mechanism, that is, with the ability to decide what should be done in particular circumstances. The higher levels of skills in the crafts and trades lie less in the ability to execute particular manual operations, such as shaping clay on a potter's wheel or using a hacksaw to cut cleanly through a piece of metal, than in deciding what shape is needed or exactly where the cut should be made. Similarly, top-level athletic skill lies in the strategy of the game rather than in the ability to make accurate strokes, and the soloist's skill transcends the mere playing of the instrument to the interpretation of the music. These high-grade aspects of what are commonly thought of as sensory-motor skills are really forms of *intellectual skill,* analogous to the skills of the administrator, manager, politician, or military officer. For all these individuals, the immediate input data and its meaning on any occasion may be perfectly clear, and the actions needed to effect their decisions may be easy. Their skill lies in the linking of perception to action implied in deciding what should be done.

It is probably fair to argue that all skills essentially involve the whole chain of central mechanisms, but that different types of tasks emphasize different links in the chain, so that when we speak of skills as "perceptual" or "motor" or "intellectual," we are classifying in relative rather than absolute terms. One must also keep in mind that skill involves action in relation to external situations, so that popularly recognized classes of skill may differ not so much in the central mechanisms involved as in the features of the external world to which they relate. Thus, manipulative skills relate to concrete objects such as tools and materials, intellectual skills relate to ideas and principles of function, and managerial and social skills relate to other people. The common feature running through them all is the deployment of capacity in a manner which becomes more efficient and effective with experience.

The improvement of performance that comes with experience does not seem to result from any increase in the individual's basic capacities, but from the efficiency with which they are used. Exercise taken in the course of physical training increases the strength and endurance of muscles, not by increasing the number of muscle fibers, but by increasing the size of the existing fibers and the blood supply to them. In the same way, experience and training in skills do not raise the number of active nerve cells in the brain—they do not increase in number after birth—but affect the extent and subtlety of their interconnections and their readiness to fire. Thus, there are limits to the effects of experience and training.

Individuals differ in their endowments of muscle fibers, brain cells, and other bodily structures, so that while experience and training can develop everyone's power to some extent, they can never be the means of achieving equality unless steps are taken actually to prevent the development of the full potentialities of the best endowed. No training, for example, can bring a severely brain-damaged person to high-grade intellectual performance, any more than a severely physically handicapped individual can be trained to run a four-minute mile.

Training and experience are nevertheless vitally important for the realization of capacities. This is especially true in the early years, during which brain and body mechanisms are maturing. Such maturation has to take place to a certain extent before particular performances are possible: for instance, muscular strength and coordination, together with balance, are necessary before a young child can begin to walk. It is often claimed that there are crucial times during the course of maturation at which, if appropriate experience is not forthcoming, ability is permanently impaired. For example, animals reared in darkness, or human beings born blind who subsequently recover their sight, seem never to attain the full subtlety of visual perception possessed by those who have seen from birth (see e.g., Gregory, 1966). Similarly, it is commonly regarded as impossible to acquire a second language perfectly to the extent of true bilingualism if it has not been learned to some extent by the age of five.

Such crucial periods are perhaps understandable when it is recognized that learning is essentially cumulative. We approach any new situation with what we have learned in the course of previous experience, and this determines the way the new situation is tackled. Doing so adds to our experience and thus modifies both the way in which we tackle any similar situation later, and our approach to any subsequent new situation. Early experiences are thus likely to have a disproportionate effect on the way in which we view events, and on the skills we bring to meet them. If, for instance, our early experience has contained a wealth of visual material and our control of movement is good, we are likely to tackle problems by means of visually guided manipulation to a greater extent than we should if our predominant experience and capacities had been of other kinds.

The practical implication is, of course, that skills developed in later stages of life, and training for them, have to link onto a long line of previous development, and that if a wide ranging potentiality for learning new skills is to be attained, early training must lay a relatively broad and generalized foundation. This is not a plea for a superficial education covering a wide range of subjects, but rather for education which gives a thorough training in the use of verbal and numerical symbols, intellectual manipulations of data and ideas, sensory-motor coordinations, and social interaction, all of which, with varying emphases, are fundamental to any effective skilled activity.

Summary

Skill lies in the use of capacities efficiently and effectively as the result of experience and practice. The study of skill has developed greatly since the 1940s from having been largely concerned with manual operations in industry, to a range of manual, athletic, intellectual, and social activities in many walks of life.

The chain of central mechanisms leading from sensory input to motor output fall into three main divisions: first, perceptual coding of incoming data; second, choice of response, or more precisely, translation from perception to response; and third, the phasing and sequencing of action. None of these stages works in a manner consistent with simple stimulus-response concepts; instead, all are concerned with more or less complex computations based upon incoming data but also incorporating influences from the previous state of the organism, both immediate and more remote, stored in separate short- and long-term memory systems. Between the first and second stages there appears to be a short-term buffer store and a "gate" which protects the second stage from interference from new data until its computations are complete and response based on them has begun.

Feedback loops within the organism, and the observation of the results of action upon external objects, make the whole system into a self-regulating servomechanism.

Paralleling the main chain from input to output is a secondary system which has diffuse arousing effects on the stages of the main chain, tending to intensify their activity at times of effort, special demand, and stress. This secondary system is associated with the autonomic nervous system, whose activity is taken as an index of this type of arousal.

The various mechanisms identified are dealt with separately in greater detail in subsequent chapters.

Types of skill, such as perceptual, intellectual, and motor, can be identified according to the stage of the central mechanisms mainly involved, although all stages appear to be involved to some extent in all skills. In each case, acquisition of skill seems not to increase basic capacities, but to improve the efficiency and effectiveness with which they are used. Learning is a cumulative process, with each new task or experience being dealt with in terms acquired in dealing with previous situations. Initial experiences and training early in life thus appear to be especially influential in laying the foundations on which the realization of potentialities can be built.

Discrimination

2

The psychological study of human performance traditionally begins with a treatment of *psychophysics*, that is, relating sensory experience to physical measures. This tradition is sound because the judgments involved in psychophysical experiments represent a form of simple *decision making* which lends itself to relatively precise measurement and mathematical formulation. Analogies of these simple decisions are found in other areas of psychological function and in the more complex decisions of everyday life, so that theories developed in the psychophysical field provide a framework for thought which can be applied far beyond the experiments upon which they are based.

Early experiments showed that psychophysical judgments were amenable to training, and therefore capable of displaying skill. For example, Volkmann (1858) examined the effects of practice on errors made in distinguishing whether one or both points of a pair of dividers, with the points close together, had been applied to the skin. He found that when the divider was applied to the tip of the left middle finger, errors in discrimination decreased with practice from about 15 percent to about 3 percent. At the same time, there was a similar improvement in discrimination by the right middle finger, without practice, but not by the left forearm. Thus, while the improved discrimination was not confined only to the member practiced, it was not completely general but was limited to those areas close to, or bilaterally symmetrical with, the practiced area. Woodworth (1938) suggested that the improvement was due to recognition by the subjects of a subtle difference in the sensations produced by one and two points, without their actually feeling two distinct points as opposed to one. In other words, judgment was based on a central effect which was not necessarily a precise copy of the objective stimulus.

Thresholds and the Weber fraction

In the nineteenth century, researchers found that amounts of sound or light that were physically measurable were not always heard or seen, even when subjects were fully alerted to detect them. To account for this observation, there developed the concept of a *threshold*, or minimum quantity, above which a stimulus had to rise in order to enter the perceptual mechanism. It was also noted early that the stimulus level required to pass this threshold was not completely fixed, but varied from instant to instant in an apparently random manner. Just why this was so was not clear, although it was reasonable to assume that the central effect of a given physical stimulus may vary from one moment to another (Cattell, 1893; Solomons, 1900; Oldfield, 1955).

The central effect of a stimulus, such as the frequency of nerve impulses generated, is commonly assumed, following Thurstone (1927a, b), to be proportional to the logarithm of the physical intensity. In other words, there is a *logarithmic transformation* between physical stimulus and central effect. Such a transformation provides what is probably the simplest explanation of the fact that the least noticeable increase in stimulus intensity is a constant fraction of the intensity from which the increase is made. This relationship, known as the *Weber fraction*, may be written

$$\frac{\delta S}{S} = \text{a constant} \tag{2.1}$$

where δS is the least noticeable increase of stimulus intensity from a given level S measured in physical units. It may also be written

$$\frac{G}{L} = \text{a constant} \tag{2.2}$$

where G and L are the greater and lesser respectively of two quantities compared, or alternatively

$$\log G - \log L = \text{a constant} \tag{2.3}$$

The implication of this last equation, taken with Thurstone's assumption, is that the discriminability of two stimuli depends upon a constant difference between their central effects.

It can be argued that this holds even though the Weber fraction is not entirely constant but rises substantially at low values of S. The rise is abolished if a constant (r) is added to S, so that in place of Equation 2.1, we write

$$\frac{\delta S}{S + r} = \text{a constant} \tag{2.4}$$

and in place of Equation 2.3,

$$\log (G + r) - \log (L + r) = \text{a constant} \tag{2.5}$$

The quantity r is small, so that it affects the Weber fraction substantially only when stimulus intensities are small, and can usually be neglected when intensities are large. The quantity r is commonly assumed to represent spontaneous activity in the sense organ and central pathways and projection areas, so that it does in a very real sense add to S.

The attempt to tie discrimination down into such central effects as frequencies of nerve impulses is plausible for simple sensory magnitudes, but may be questionable for more complex perceptual quantities such as lengths of lines or numbers of objects. Such quantities must, however, somehow be represented centrally, so that although the precise mode of representation is not clear, treating perceptual magnitudes in this way is not unjustified.

The signal detection theory

It used to be assumed that if the threshold was not passed but subjects nevertheless had to respond, they guessed at random. There were, however, two facts which called this idea into question. The first was that the measured threshold depended very much upon the degree of confidence required of the subjects: their thresholds were higher if they had to report a signal only when sure than if they could do so even when somewhat doubtful. The second fact was that if subjects were not sure but were nevertheless forced to guess whether a signal had been given or not, guesses over a number of trials were substantially better than chance, implying that the signal had been perceived to some extent even though the subjects had little or no confidence that it had occurred.

Currently, the method generally accepted to account for these facts is the *signal detection theory* developed by Tanner, Swets, and their associates, working on the detection of faint sounds against background noise, or faint visual signals on an illuminated background in which slight random variations constitute "visual noise" (Tanner & Swets, 1954; Swets et al., 1961; Green & Swets, 1966; McNicol, 1972).

In these investigations, a basic research situation is one in which the subject is given a series of trials. In each trial there is a brief presentation of either the background noise plus a signal, or the background noise alone. The subject's task is to decide whether or not a signal was present. Researchers argue that during each presentation the subject observes a quantity x which, because of the noise, is liable to vary randomly in magnitude from trial to trial. We can represent the magnitude of x observed over a series of trials in which no signal was present by a distribution such as that shown for *Noise Alone* in Figure 2.1. The noise may be either *external* due to variability of the stimulation presented to the subject, or *internal* due to randomness

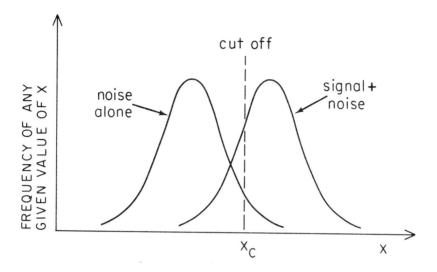

Figure 2.1. *The basic signal detection model.*

in the activity of the sense organ, neural pathways, and brain, as already represented by *r* in Equations 2.4 and 2.5. The shape of the noise distribution will depend on the distributions of the various components making up the noise and on any transformations of physical quantities that take place in the sense organs or the brain, but for the purpose of our present discussion it can be tentatively regarded as normal.

The quantity *x* for presentations in which a signal is present is assumed to have a similar distribution to the noise, but with each observation increased by the amount of the signal, as shown in the *Signal + Noise* curve of Figure 2.1. The subject is assumed to establish a cutoff point x_c and to treat any level of *x* above this point as *Signal*, and any point below it as *Noise Alone* or *No Signal*. If the signals are strong enough for the distributions to be well separated, the discrimination of *Signal* from *No Signal* can be virtually complete. If, however, the signal strength is weaker, so that there is overlap between the distributions, discrimination cannot always be accurate. Part of one or the other distribution or of both will inevitably be on the wrong side of x_c so that errors will be made.

The model represented in Figure 2.1 treats discrimination in terms of two parameters, d' and β. The former, d', is the distance between corresponding points—say, the means—of the two curves measured in standard deviation units. We can thus write

$$d' = \frac{\bar{X}_S - \bar{X}_N}{\sigma} \tag{2.6}$$

where $\bar{X}_S$ is the mean of the *Signal + Noise* curve and $\bar{X}_N$ the mean of *Noise Alone* curve and σ is the standard deviation.

The second parameter, β, is the *likelihood ratio* that a central effect of the magnitude represented by x_c is due to *Signal + Noise* as opposed to *Noise Alone*. In other words, it is the ratio of the frequencies (f)—that is, the heights of the ordinates—at x_c, so that we write

$$\beta = \frac{f_S}{f_N} \text{ at } x_c \tag{2.7}$$

If the distributions of *Signal + Noise* and *Noise Alone* are known or can be assumed, d' and β can be calculated from the proportions of the two possible classes of correct response thus:

(a) *Yes*, when a signal is present—represented by the area of the *Signal + Noise* distribution to the right of x_c in Figure 2.1.
(b) *No*, when a signal is not present—represented by the area of the *Noise Alone* distribution to the left of x_c.

If, for example, the distributions are normal, the distance from x_c to the mean of the *Signal + Noise* distribution measured in standard deviation units can be found from a table of the normal probability integral by noting the deviation required to produce the proportion of (a) responses. Similarly, the distance from x_c to the mean of the *Noise Alone* distribution can be found by noting the deviation required to produce the proportion of (b) responses. Assuming the two distributions are of equal variance, the value of d' will be the sum of these two deviations. For instance, if the proportions of (a) and (b) are .90 and .95, the two deviations would be 1.28 and 1.64 respectively, and d' would be 2.92.

The same result could have been obtained using the proportions of the two possible classes of error:

(c) *Misses*—that is, responses of *no* when a signal is in fact present, represented by the area of the *Signal + Noise* distribution to the left of x_c.
(d) *False positives*—that is, replies of *yes* when no signal is present, represented by the area of the *Noise Alone* distribution to the right of x_c.

The value of β can be calculated, when the distributions are normal, from a table of the ordinates of a normal distribution. For the example just quoted, these are .176 and .103 respectively, so that $\beta = 1.71$. The value of β diminishes as x_c is moved to the left.

A table to find d' and β for different values of (c) and (d) responses is given in the Appendix.

The value of d' is the measure of true discriminability in terms of the ratio between signal strength and the variability of the noise level. β, as a measure of the cutoff point x_c, can be thought of as expressing the extent of any bias towards one response or the other. In the situation we are considering, it will indicate the confidence with which judgments are made. For example, a large value of β, implying a high cutoff well to the right in Figure 2.1, means that the subject is biasing responses towards *no*, or in other words, demanding a high degree of confidence before saying *yes*. As a result, the proportion of *yes* responses will be relatively low and the proportion of *no* responses will be correspondingly high, while among the errors made there will be few false positives and a relatively large number of misses. The subject is able to make judgments in terms of more than one cutoff by defining different levels of confidence such as "Sure; Not quite sure; Uncertain; Not quite sure not; Sure not." The proportion of misses will decrease and of false positives will increase from the first category to the last.

What is *X*?

The advocates of the signal detection theory have stressed that much of its usefulness does not depend on being able to specify the quantity X which the observer uses as a basis for decisions. It is commonly assumed that X is a linear function of central activity in the brain. If this is so, however, the distributions cannot possibly be normal and are probably of unequal variance. They cannot, for example, extend from minus infinity to plus infinity as strictly normal distributions would, but extend instead from zero to some maximum set by the capacity of the brain mechanism concerned. If the noise is conceived as consisting of random neural impulses occurring within a brief period of time, the response distributions would be approximately of Poisson form, with a variance equal to the mean, and would look like those shown in Figure 2.2. Calculations in terms of normal distributions and equal variances may nevertheless remain valid (Tanner & Swets, 1954).

All our discussion so far has been in terms of the proportions of the four possible responses—*yes* or *no* when a signal either was or was not present. These proportions would remain the same if the measure along the X axis was transformed, as, for example, by plotting not the number of neural impulses, but the logarithm of the number. We are thus in the position

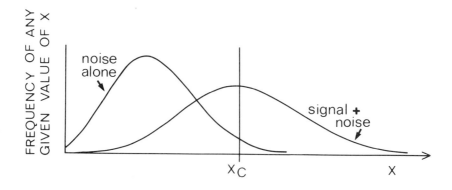

Figure 2.2. *The basic signal detection model assuming Poisson-like distributions.*

of an experimenter who wishes to perform an analysis of variance on data with nonnormal distributions and unequal variances, and can follow the procedure recommended in that case of transforming the measure so as to make the distributions normal and the variances equal. Doing this will in no way invalidate the test or, in our case, the computation of d', and as long as we work in terms of our four proportions, we do not need to specify what transformation of the X axis has been made.

Placing the cutoff point

Setting the point of cutoff is to some extent under the subject's voluntary control, and there seems clearly to be scope for the exercise of skill in doing so. The objectively optimum point can be calculated if the rewards attached to each of the correct responses and the costs of the two types of error are known and are measurable in the same units:

$$\text{Optimum } \beta = \frac{\text{Probability of } No \ signal}{\text{Probability of } Signal} \quad (2.8)$$

$$\times \ \frac{\text{Value of correct } no + \text{Cost of incorrect } yes}{\text{Value of correct } yes + \text{Cost of incorrect } no}$$

In order to fix the cutoff optimally, however, the subject needs to know or be able to assess all these quantities, and also to relate them together. The evidence from a number of experiments on discrimination (e.g., Ulehla, 1966) and on guessing and betting (e.g., Edwards, 1961) makes it clear that the optimum is seldom if ever achieved. At least part of the reason probably lies in the fact that the limited span of short-term retention makes it impossible to assess accurately the way in which sequences of signals have been constructed: subjects tend to give undue weight at each point in the series to the three or four items just presented. Another part of the reason may lie in a noticeable tendency to overestimate the probability of rare events and underestimate that of frequent ones (Howard, 1963). Still more of the explanation may lie in the inability of subjects to adjust their strategies to evaluate values and costs completely. For example, Pitz and Downing (1967), in a guessing task, found that performance was near optimum when the values of different guesses were equal, but departed markedly from optimum when they were not.

Knowledge and experience of the signal sequences, rewards, and punishments can, however, affect the setting of cutoff points to some extent (e.g., Taub & Myers, 1961; Katz, 1964). For example, Laming (1962) required his subjects to sort packs of cards into two piles according to whether they carried a longer or shorter line. He found that when the two lengths did not appear with equal frequency, subjects adjusted their cutoff points in a way that reduced the errors made in responding to the more frequent signal. Similar adjustments result from incentives. For instance, Swets and Sewall (1963), using a task in which subjects detected tones in short bursts of noise, showed that offering monetary rewards for improved performance affected β but left d' unchanged.

In the absence of any knowledge of the signal sequence or other considerations, subjects must base their setting of cutoff points on their knowledge of the noise distribution alone. When doing this they presumably set a level which will give a tolerable—usually very low—likelihood of making false positive responses.

Absolute judgments

The model of Figure 2.1 can logically be extended to cover absolute judgments in which stimuli such as weights must be classed into categories of heaviness, or sounded tones into categories of loudness or pitch. The simplest case is that in which one of two quantities is presented in any trial, and the subject must say whether it is the greater or the lesser. In this case, Figure 2.1 remains valid if the distributions of *Signal + Noise* and *Noise Alone* are relabeled *Greater Signal + Noise* and *Lesser Signal + Noise* respectively. Equation 2.6 also still applies if $\bar{X}_G$ and $\bar{X}_L$—the means of the greater and lesser quantities—are substituted for $\bar{X}_S$ and $\bar{X}_N$.

When there are more than two possible signals, the stimuli can be envisaged as producing distributions along a "decision axis" on which there are several cutoff points dividing each category of response from the next, as shown in Figure 2.3. It can be seen that each category covers a band of magnitudes of signal-plus-noise.

Several studies have shown that the number of clearly distinguishable categories in tasks of this kind is, for most people, severely limited, and that if finer categorization is called for, misclassifications occur. For example, Pollack (1952), who required subjects to assign numbers to tones of varying pitches equidistant on a logarithmic scale ranging from 100 to 8,000 cps, found that only about five or six classes could be reliably distinguished. Again, Miller (1956) has surveyed data which indicates that comparatively small numbers of distinguishable classes are also found for judgments of other quantities such as loudness (about six) and points on a line (about nine).

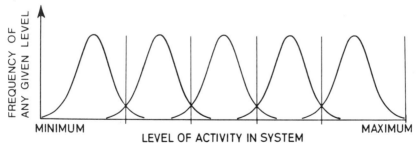

Figure 2.3. Extension of the signal detection model to cases where absolute judgments are required of several values of a variable quantity.

It is clear that the distributions shown in Figure 2.3 are of amounts of activity in the system which range from a level which is indistinguishable from noise up to some maximum which represents saturation. If so, the number of discriminable classes will be the number of signal-plus-noise distributions that can be fitted in between minimum and maximum with acceptably low overlap. This, however, is clearly not the source of the severe limitation found by Pollack and in the studies surveyed by Miller. If it were, discriminability would depend on the total range of stimuli that can be perceived, and would be independent of the range actually presented. Pollack (1952, 1953a) has shown that this is not so: the number of discriminable pitches remains about the same whether the stimuli are presented over a wide range of frequencies or concentrated within a narrow one. The same is true whether the frequencies are all near one or the other end of the range. Similar results have been obtained for different loudness levels (Hodge & Pollack, 1962).

The implication is that the limitation lies in the decision process rather than in the range of stimuli. The range over which decision is made—the decision axis—is limited but is capable of adjustment, either to cover a wide range of stimuli, or to "focus down" upon a narrower range. How this is done is not clear, but one possibility is to assume first, as we have already done, that central effect is proportional to the logarithm of the physical stimulus.

We then make a second assumption that the signal can be attenuated either before or after the logarithmic transformation of the data has taken place. Attenuation before the transformation would essentially subtract a constant amount from log S, and different levels of attenuation would produce a series of relationships between log S and its central effect as shown in Figure 2.4A. The effect would be to determine the *portion* of the total range

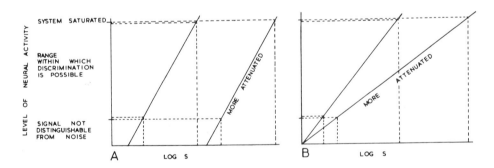

Figure 2.4. Effects on the decision axis of attenuating the signal before and after a logarithmic transformation of data. The effect of attenuation before logarithmic transformation is shown in A. In this case the effect of attenuation is to increase the absolute values of log S over which discrimination can be made while the range of values remains unaffected. The effect of attenuation after logarithmic transformation is shown in B. In this case the main effect of attenuation is to increase the range of values of log S over which discrimination can be made.

of stimuli over which the decision mechanism operated, without affecting its extent—for example, it might shift from low pitches to high. Attenuation after the logarithmic transformation of the data would alter the slope of the relation between log S and its central effect as shown in Figure 2.4B, and would affect the *range* over which the decision mechanism operated. For example, attenuation would determine whether discriminative capacity was spread over a wide range of pitches from high to low or was confined to one part of the scale.

The limited number of classes obtainable on the decision axis implies that the cutoffs are not, in fact, fixed points as shown in Figure 2.3, but are subject to substantial fluctuation from moment to moment. For many purposes this fluctuation does not have to be distinguished from variation in the signal and noise, so that a diagram such as Figure 2.1 can conveniently represent the situation even if the distributions include random fluctuation of the criterion point as well as noise in the signal, sense organs, and perceptual mechanism. In this case, however, the distinction must be made. The situation envisaged is shown in Figure 2.5: the number of discriminable categories is limited essentially by the distributions of the criteria, and this holds whether the decision axis is spread over a wide range of stimuli as in Figure 2.5A, or focused on a narrower range as in Figure 2.5B.

The decision axis tends to adjust rapidly to the range of stimuli presented (Tresselt & Volkmann, 1942). It is clear from Figure 2.5 that if the stimuli cover the whole range of the decision axis equally, discrimination will be most efficient when the cutoffs are equally spaced. There is some evidence

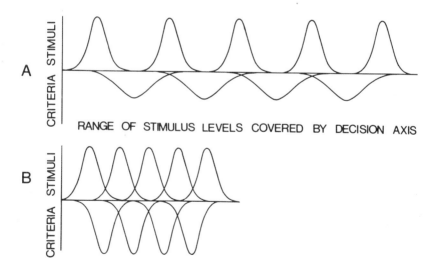

Figure 2.5. Modification of Figure 2.3, providing distributions of cutoff points as well as of signals, over two ranges of stimuli: A, wide; B, narrower.

that this tends to occur even when the stimuli are concentrated in parts of the range. For example, Sherif et al. (1958) presented subjects with a series of six weights ranging from 55–141g in random order, and obtained the results shown at the top of Figure 2.6. They then presented weights in pairs, first the one represented by the "anchor" in Figure 2.6, and then one of the original six. As the anchor became heavier, all the other weights tended to be classed into the lighter categories. The heavy anchor had stretched the range covered by the decision axis and thus broadened the range of weights included in the lighter categories.

The pileup of judgments in the heavier categories with the 141g anchor is surprising, but several other studies (e.g., John, 1973, 1975) have also shown clearly that stimuli tend to be judged as more similar to immediately preceding stimuli than they really are. Why this should occur is not wholly clear, but the results of a large number of experiments seem to be consistent with the operation of two opposing tendencies: (1) a spontaneous tendency

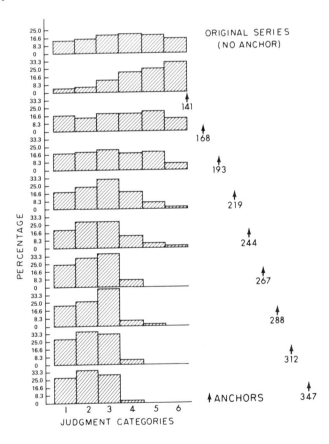

Figure 2.6. *Categories in which a series of six weights were judged without an "anchor" (top) and with "anchors" heavier by increasing amounts.*

for the range over which the decision axis is deployed to shrink, or to be focused down more closely, so that stimuli at both ends tend to be judged as more extreme than they actually are, and (2) a tendency for the identification of a stimulus to expand the range of the decision axis from the point at which it is identified.

Thus, identification of a stimulus as "large"—say 9 on a 10-point scale—would expand the widths of the categories towards the smaller end, so that if the next stimulus is less than 9, it will be judged as larger than it would otherwise be. Similarly, a stimulus identified as, say, 2 would tend to lead to a subsequent larger stimulus being identified as smaller than it should be. John (1975) has produced evidence that, in a series of presentations, these tendencies are reduced as the intervals between stimuli are lengthened. This finding appears to imply that the expansion of the range of the decision axis is temporary, and that the axis shrinks again with lapse of time after the judgment is made.

Skill in making absolute judgments is shown by the fact that the number of categories of identification can be increased with practice. The example most studied has been that of "absolute pitch"—the ability to recognize reliably a number of pitches far in excess of the five attained by Pollack's subjects. Several early writers believed that absolute pitch was an inherited ability, but experimental studies have clearly shown that it can be acquired, or at least very greatly improved, with training (for a review see Neu, 1947). Identification in such cases is usually in terms of some familiar labeling, such as the musical scale. The ability to identify pitch tends to be better for notes produced by a musical instrument or for a timbre familiar to the subject. Effectiveness of training depends on the extent to which the trainee's attention is engaged: active attempts to sing notes of specified pitches are a more effective means of training than passive attempts at identification.

It seems clear that judgments of pitch are made in terms of a scale held in the memory with which each incoming note is compared, and that the skill of absolute pitch means that a scale has been built up which is more detailed, and perhaps more readily available for use, than is normal. It must also, presumably, be sufficiently firmly established to resist the subtle shifts which result from moment-to-moment focusing of the decision axis and the effects of preceding stimuli.

Something of the nature of such scales is indicated in the report of a subject studied by Carpenter (1951). This subject identified pitches by a two-fold operation: first the note on the scale, such as A-flat or C-sharp, and then the octave, often after some hesitation. Carpenter noted that this accords with Bachem's (1948) view that the judgment of "chroma," by which he meant position in the octave, is different from "tone height," that is, frequency in terms of octaves. We can, perhaps, see that the ability to recognize melodic intervals, which is associated but not identical with ability to identify pitch, could represent the first of these qualities without the second (Rowe & Ivinskis, 1972).

Skills analogous to absolute pitch seem to be found in most activities which require the continual making of fine discriminations, such as those made by dyers in distinguishing subtle shades of color or by steelworkers who must decide on the basis of color when molten metal is ready to be poured into casting molds. Examples from other senses include the fine tactile discrimination shown by workers who grade wool and other fibers, the pressure discrimination by cheese graders to assess softness, and the sensitivity of "palate" displayed by wine tasters. These skills have been studied less than has absolute pitch, perhaps because in many cases human workers are being replaced by measuring instruments. They constitute, however, skills whose acquisition and use is of obvious theoretical interest, and will probably have practical application for some time to come.

Comparative judgments

The discriminations discussed so far have all been of quantities presented one at a time. Much finer discriminations are obtainable when two quantities to be distinguished from each other are presented either together or almost together. A possible reason for the greater accuracy may be that when both quantities are presented simultaneously, the decision axis can be focused onto a narrower range than when only one quantity is presented at a time.

If the noise affecting both signals fluctuated from moment to moment in exactly the same way, Equation 2.6 would continue to hold, with $\bar{X}_G$ and $\bar{X}_L$ substituted for $\bar{X}_S$ and $\bar{X}_N$. Experimental evidence suggests, however, that the noise affecting the two signals varies independently, so that in place of Equation 2.6 we write

$$d' = \frac{\bar{X}_G - \bar{X}_L}{\sqrt{\sigma_G^2 + \sigma_L^2}} = \frac{\bar{X}_{(G-L)}}{\sigma_{(G-L)}} \tag{2.9}$$

where $\bar{X}_G$ and $\bar{X}_L$ are, as before, the means of the greater and lesser stimuli, G and L, σ_G and σ_L, are the standard deviations of their distributions, $\bar{X}_{(G-L)}$ is the mean difference between the greater and lesser stimuli, and $\sigma_{(G-L)}$ is the standard deviation of this difference.

The type of judgment demanded differs from that of the absolute case. Instead of having to say "Yes, a stimulus was present" or "No, it was not," or to put a stimulus into a category, the subject has to indicate whether, say, the stimulus A presented on the right is greater than B presented on the left, or vice versa. The statement "A is greater than B" will include correct answers when A is objectively greater than B, and incorrect answers when it is not. Similarly, the statement "B is greater than A" will include correct answers when B is objectively greater than A, and incorrect answers when it is not. In these circumstances, a measure of confidence in terms of β is not possible. A measure of confidence can be obtained, however, if the subject is allowed to say "A is equal to B" since greater confidence will lead to lower proportions of equal judgments. An additional method, obtainable under certain conditions, will be discussed later.

The effects of training and practice on comparative judgments seem to have attracted relatively little research, but it is clear that, in practical situations, experience can refine comparative judgments just as it can absolute. For example, an experienced dyer or dealer in textiles will often observe fine shades of difference in colors which most people would fail to notice. On a more complex level, expert observers can often detect subtle differences between what are, to the untrained eye, identical objects.

Inspection time and discrimination accuracy

The cases considered in this chapter so far have been of situations in which, typically, the stimuli to be judged have been presented briefly and the judgments made after the stimuli have been removed. More accurate discrimination is possible if the stimuli are presented for longer periods or until subjects give their judgments.

Several attempts have been made to formulate the effects of longer inspection time on the accuracy of discrimination, in ways which broadly follow the signal detection model. Early studies sought some formulation which would make discriminability rise continuously with the length of time spent inspecting the display. These studies have been summarized by the author (Welford, 1960b, 1968), who found that no single formulation accounted for all the available experimental results. Discriminability appeared not to rise continuously, but to do so for a time and then to flatten out, so that however much longer time was taken, no improvement of accuracy resulted after a certain point. Some newer and more successful approaches have been summarized and discussed by Vickers (1970) and Pike (1973).

These more recent approaches are based on the fact that when the distributions of the two quantities A and B shown to the subject overlap, as they obviously will in experiments on fine discrimination, the differences between them $(X_A - X_B)$ at any instant will sometimes be positive and sometimes negative, as shown in Figure 2.7. The subject is assumed to take a series of brief samples of the data, and to accumulate the results until some criterion for A > B or B > A is reached, when he will make a decision accordingly.

The accumulator model

The theory which appears to fit the facts best is that of Vickers' *accumulator model*. According to this model, the subject is assumed to accumulate the quantities by which X_A differs from X_B in two separate stores, one for which $X_A > X_B$ and one for which $X_B > X_A$. This is done until the total in one or the other store reaches a criterion value at which time

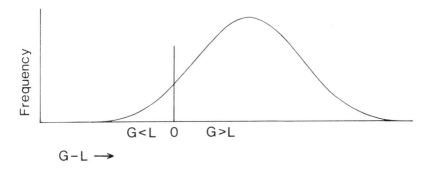

Figure 2.7. *Distribution of differences between two closely similar quantities, the greater G and the lesser L, both independently disturbed by random noise.*

the subject makes a decision either that A > B or vice versa. This process is illustrated in Figure 2.8. A decision A > B will, of course, be correct if A = *G* and incorrect if A = *L*, and similarly a decision B > A will be correct if B = *G* and incorrect if B = *L*.

Reaction time will depend on the number of samples that have to be placed in *both* stores before the total in one or other reaches criterion. Thus if *G* and *L* are very different, almost all the samples are likely to go into the store corresponding to $X_G > X_L$ and the size of each will be large, so that the criterion will be reached quickly, and reaction time for a correct

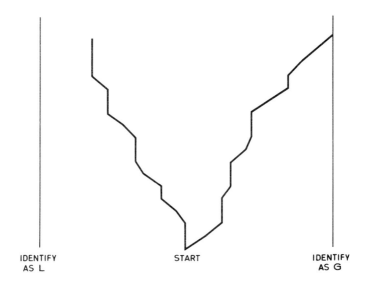

Figure 2.8 *The process of discrimination envisaged in Vickers' accumulator model.*

response will be short. When there is less difference between G and L, the samples will be smaller and some are likely to go to the store for $X_L > X_G$ before the criterion value is reached. Reaction time for a correct response will therefore be longer than when G and L are very different.

Reaction times for errors will tend to be longer than for correct responses, although if the criterion is low, one or two chance samples in close proximity with $X_L >> X_G$ might lead to an error being made with a relatively short reaction time. Vickers (1970), in experiments where subjects had to decide which of two lines presented side by side was the longer, has in fact shown that the time taken for errors tends to rise as the criterion values become higher.

The accumulator model accounts neatly for the fact that however fine the discrimination required, it cannot be improved indefinitely by increased decision time. It is obvious from Figure 2.7 that, even if A and B were objectively equal, X_A and X_B would often differ substantially at any one instant, so that appreciable quantities would be fed into the two stores. One or the other store would thus be brought to criterion in a time not much longer than would be required when A and B differed appreciably.

The accumulator model can also explain some other perceptual phenomena. For example, Vickers (1972) has shown that this approach can cover the main facts of perceptual alternation seen in such well-known ambiguous figures as the Rubin vase-face diagram and the Schroeder staircase. Vickers considered the designs shown in Figure 2.9, each of which subjects tend to see sometimes as a white cross on a black background, and sometimes as a black cross on a white background. The predominant tendency is to see the narrower sectors as forming the cross. Vickers suggested that the central effects of the sectors varied in width randomly from moment to moment, and that on first viewing the design, the subject accumulates samples of White <

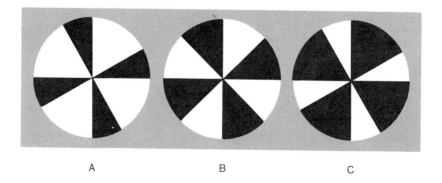

A   B   C

Figure 2.9. *Three Maltese cross patterns, in which the main factor influencing figure-ground differentiation is the relative sizes of the black and the white sector angles. The crosslike configuration with the smaller angle tends to be seen as a figure, as in a or c, while the equal sector angles in b give rise to two equally probable responses.*

Black and of Black < White in two stores until one, say White < Black, reaches criterion and the appropriate sectors appear as the cross. The subject repeats the process until criterion is again reached. If it is the same criterion of White < Black, as before, no change of percept occurs, but if the other criterion of Black < White is reached, the percept suddenly changes. This process is assumed to go on being repeated as long as the subject looks at the design.

If this account is correct, three results should follow, all of which are supported by experimental findings:

(a) The percept which predominates should tend to be the same as the one which appears first.
(b) The alternation should not be entirely under voluntary control, although it could be controlled to some extent by setting the criteria. If the criteria were low, alternation would tend to be more rapid than if they were higher. Several experiments have shown that subjects can slow down or speed up alternation at will, but cannot prevent it entirely.
(c) The durations of the two percepts should be more nearly equal if the sectors are objectively equal than if they are not. Similarly, in more complex designs, the durations of the percepts should vary with their probability.

Vickers' suggestions were based on the findings of several previous reseachers, especially those summarized by Sadler and Mefford (1970). His suggestions have been confirmed experimentally by Nettelbeck (1973a), using the Necker cube (see Figure 3.2A).

Susceptibility to training
The accumulator model depends essentially upon three parameters:

(a) time per sample, or as Vickers has termed it, *inspection time*;
(b) random variability of the quantities to be distinguished, that is *noise* as defined in signal detection theory, either external in the stimulus or internal in the subjects' sense organs, pathways, and central mechanisms; and
(c) *caution*, as implied by the level at which criteria are set.

It is pertinent to ask here which discrimination processes are subject to training and are therefore to be regarded as parameters of skill, and which are facets of basic capacity unchanged by training or experience. Experimental work done so far does not provide definite answers to these questions, but strong indications are contained in results obtained by Nettelbeck (Vickers et al., 1972; Nettelbeck, 1973a), who measured the three parameters separately and examined their stability in individuals from one situation to another.

Inspection time was measured by using two vertical lines side by side which were sufficiently different from each other—in the ratio of 4 to 3—for them to be discriminated accurately in one inspection time. They were shown for intervals ranging from 12 to 120 msec. At the end of the exposure time, both lines were immediately extended so that subjects could not obtain further data from afterimages or other effects of the stimulus continuing after exposure had ceased. Accuracy rose asymptotically towards 100 percent as the exposure time increased. In order to allow for the errors inevitable even with very easy discrimination, accuracy was regarded as having reached asymptote at 97.5 percent, and the exposure at which this level was reached was taken as the measure of inspection time. Inspection time of the ten subjects in this study ranged from 85 to 169 msec, with a mean of 106. This measure appeared stable, since a separate determination of inspection time with the same subjects gave a range from 74 to 144 msec, with a mean of 107 and a product-moment correlation between the two sets of individual times of +.80. A second group of ten subjects gave a range from 74 to 156 msec, with a mean of 101.

Noise was measured by giving, under conditions similar to the foregoing, pairs of lines providing discriminations from easy to very fine at an exposure of 100 msec, which was taken as a rough average measure of inspection time. Cumulative normal curves were fitted to the percentages of correct responses plotted against differences of line length, and the standard deviations of these curves were used to derive measures of noise. Individual estimates of noise ranged from .19 to .32 degrees of visual angle, with a mean of .23. The measures obtained by individual subjects in two different runs of the experiment were found to have a product-moment correlation of +.87, indicating that the measure of noise, like that of inspection time, was stable. Noise appeared to be independent of inspection time, implying that they constituted different individual characteristics.

Some indication of caution is obtained from reaction time. If we put λ for inspection time, then

$$\text{Reaction time} = a + b\lambda \qquad (2.10)$$

where a is a constant concerned with the choice and execution of the response and b is the number of samples (inspections) required before a criterion is reached. For any given fineness of discrimination, increasing caution will lead to a rise in b. A somewhat more refined measure of caution is the slope of the function relating reaction time to fineness of discrimination. Nettelbeck found that the reaction times of individual subjects showed correlations ranging from +.47 to +.74 between two different experimental sessions, indicating that they were fairly stable measures, although less so than inspection time and noise.

As expected, reaction times correlated negatively with errors. Correlation with inspection times was low, indicating, perhaps, that of those individuals with long inspection times some collect data slowly, while others collect data more rapidly but continue doing so until they reach higher criteria of accuracy. Reaction times understandably correlated more highly with noise: individuals whose noise level is high need to adopt high criteria if their performance is to be accurate.

Presentation of the stimuli for 100 msec followed by the *backward masking* achieved by the immediate lengthening of the lines, confines the data to approximately one inspection time. Without the backward masking, aftereffects or *iconic* storage of the stimuli seem able to provide additional data for a fraction of a second. If these data can be used, the noise in the original presentation and in the stored data can be averaged, so that the measured noise level without the backward masking will be less than with it. Nettelbeck proposed that the difference between the two measurements of noise could be taken as a measure of the use made by the subject of iconic storage. He found that this measure differed substantially between individual subjects.

Nettelbeck also found that inspection time, noise, and the use of iconic storage were all related to personality test scores, as would be expected if they were indicators of basic capacities or of deeply ingrained individual characteristics. The relationships were, however, somewhat complex and will be discussed further in Chapter 8. Noise correlated negatively with scores on an intelligence test—showing again that noise tends to indicate a basic capacity or characteristic. Noise increased when subjects were subjected to strong, unpredictable electric shocks at intervals during the experimental session in which it was measured, but there was no evidence of a concurrent change of caution (Nettelbeck, 1972). Unlike the other measures, reaction time did, however, decrease with practice, suggesting that as the task became more familiar, subjects adopted somewhat lower criteria or arrived at a more efficient balance between speed and accuracy.

More work needs to be done to evaluate these measures and to determine the extents to which they are affected by training. The evidence obtained so far suggests, however, that effects of training and indications of skill in the very simple tasks studied by Vickers and Nettelbeck, must be sought in the degree of caution exercised rather than in the other measures they took. With more complex tasks, other considerations appear to arise which greatly extend the scope for skill. We shall turn to these considerations in the next chapter.

Summary

Simple judgments of magnitude and other sensory qualities provide a convenient method of studying elementary decision processes. Early studies showed that the least noticeable difference of magnitude tends to be a constant proportion of the original magnitude—the so-called Weber fraction. This relationship is most simply explained by assuming that the central effect of a stimulus is proportional to the logarithm of its magnitude, and that discriminability depends upon the difference between the central effects of stimuli.

In terms of the signal detection model, the subject has the task of distinguishing incoming signals from random activity or "noise," either in external stimuli or in the sensory pathways and brain. The model provides measures of detectability in terms of signal-to-noise ratio, and of bias in giving responses. The latter can be regarded as an indication of the degree of confidence required for a response to be given. Skill appears to be shown in such simple judgments mainly in the biasing of responses in ways which increase either accuracy or "payoff" when rewards or penalties are given for different types of correct response and error.

The signal detection theory approach can be extended from absolute detection situations to judgments of magnitude either on an absolute scale or in comparison with other magnitudes. The number of different magnitudes that can be distinguished in absolute terms is usually small, but the range of stimulation over which this number can be spread is capable of wide adjustment. Skill has been demonstrated in both absolute and comparative tasks, especially the former in which practice and experience can greatly increase the number of distinguishable categories. Examples of such skill are the "absolute pitch" possessed by many musicians, and the fine visual discrimination of color by dyers and those who deal with colored textiles.

The time taken for discrimination between two magnitudes, A and B, is well accounted for by the accumulator model which assumes that both quantities are disturbed by noise, so that when they are closely similar, their fluctuations may make the one which is objectively larger appear instantaneously smaller. The observer is assumed to take samples of data and to accumulate them in two stores, one for samples when $A > B$ and the other for samples when $B > A$. A decision is made when the total in either store reaches a criterion value. The model yields four parameters: inspection time, that is, the time required for each sample to be taken; noise; reaction time, the length of which can be taken as an indicator of degree of caution; and the extent to which data can be used from iconic storage when the stimulus has been removed. All these measures have shown substantial differences between individuals. Only reaction time showed appreciable effects of practice. This model is capable of explaining a considerable range of complex perceptual phenomena such as the alternations in the appearance of ambiguous figures.

Perceptual coding

3

It is well known that far more data are transmitted by our sense organs to the brain than we in fact perceive. It is also obvious—so obvious that its importance is often overlooked—that the data we do perceive are grouped and ordered, or, as it is termed, "coded." Thus, as regards vision, we "see" only a part of the data our eyes provide, and we see it not as a mosaic of more and less stimulated points, but as coherent objects which have form and structure as wholes. The net result of both the selection and the integration involved is an *economy* in handling sensory data, in the sense that fewer "units" are dealt with and the number of items upon which decisions have to be taken is thereby reduced.

What constitute "units" or "items" in this context is not easy to say. The attempt to specify them has been the aim of a substantial line of research which began in Europe during the second and third decades of the present century, and led to several developments, notably the studies by the *Gestalt* school of those simple, closed, regular, or symmetrical forms which seemed to be most spontaneously and easily perceived. More recently, the development both of information theory and the type of analysis involved in computer programming has given rise to attempts to reformulate the problems in mathematical terms.

The processes of selection and integration are usually closely related. The ordering of data involved in perceiving an object implies a kind of selection in which attention is directed principally to certain data while the rest are relegated to a "background" which is largely ignored and usually cannot be reported in much detail. At the same time, conscious or deliberate selection often depends on how data are organized. It can be very difficult, for example, to see a simple shape embedded in a more complex design. Again, in tasks where one type of item has to be selected from among others, ease of selection frequently depends on context. For instance, if the letter *e* has to be cancelled throughout a paragraph of prose, it is more likely to be detected in those words where it would normally be pronounced than when it would be silent (Corcoran, 1966, 1967a; Corcoran & Weening, 1968).

For convenience, however, we shall discuss selection and integration separately before looking at some general implications of both together. Since much of the evidence has already been surveyed elsewhere (e.g., Egeth, 1967; Welford, 1968), we shall look here only at certain broad principles and note some recent trends which appear to be of both theoretical and practical interest.

Selection and identification

The basis of selection

Selection can be made relatively easily in terms of certain sensory qualities. In other words, whole classes of incoming data can be filtered off at an early stage of the perceptual process. Evidence for this comes mainly from experiments on listening in which subjects presented with two messages must respond to one while ignoring the other. It has been found that selection is facilitated if one message is given in a man's voice and the other in a woman's; if one message is louder than the other; if the voices come from different sides or appear to do so because of stereophonic imbalance; or if the "wanted" message is fed into one ear and the unwanted into the other (see Broadbent, 1958; Treisman, 1960, 1964b). Evidence of this kind implies that selection can be based not only on simple sensory qualities, such as pitch or intensity or difference of sense organ, but also on more subtle distinctions, such as the differences of phase and intensity at the two ears of the subject.

Selection appears also to be facilitated by semantic differences as, for example, when one message is a passage from a novel and one from a textbook, or when messages are in different languages, or when one is sense and the other nonsense (Treisman, 1964a). Just how much the differentiation of data in these cases is based on truly semantic grounds, and how much is in terms of subtleties of rhythm or phonetic quality, is not certain.

Over and above these factors, however, selection usually seems to be made in terms of attitudes and hypotheses brought to an existing situation from past experience—that is, we tend to perceive what is familiar and what we expect to occur. It seems clear, therefore, that selection must often be a highly complex process, involving data which have already been processed to a substantial extent by the mechanisms of perception. This may well be true even when selection appears to be based on simple sensory qualities.

Results of selection

There is a substantial amount of evidence, again mainly from studies of selective listening, that reception of the signals from an "unwanted" message is in some very real way impaired. The obvious assumption is that the signal of an unwanted message is weakened, and this is supported by the fact that the electrical potentials evoked in the cortex of the brain by incoming stimuli are diminished when attention is directed away from them (Wilkinson, 1967).

Broadbent (1958) had originally assumed that the unwanted channel was completely blocked, but several experiments have now shown that this does not occur (e.g., Moray, 1959; Treisman, 1960; Treisman & Geffen, 1967). When a subject receives two messages through headphones, one message to each ear, and must pay attention to one while ignoring the other, occasional items from the ignored message will, nonetheless, be perceived. These items are especially likely to get through if they are appropriate or relevant to the wanted message at the moment they occur, or if they have special significance to the subject, such as the person's own name. Occasional "wanted" items played to the unattended ear can be detected better if they are readily discriminable, as when they are spoken in a different voice (Treisman & Riley, 1969), or are "pips" interspersed during a passage of prose (Lawson, 1966).

Looking at selectivity in more general terms, Wachtel (1967) presented evidence which suggests that attention can be conceived of as a beam of light which is focused more or less sharply on particular sources of incoming data—a concept in many ways similar to the focusing discussed in the previous chapter. He suggested that a distinction can be drawn between the narrowness of the focus at any one time, and the extent to which the beam ranges over the field at different times. He proposed that characteristic tendencies in these two respects can be regarded as facets of personality varying from one individual, or type of individual, to another. For example, the behavior of highly anxious people may be compared to a narrow beam which roams widely over the field, so that attention skips rapidly from item to item but is intensely directed to any item on which it is actually resting.

Costs of selection

A wide variety of experimental studies have made it clear that perceptual selection is a task which involves some mental activity or "work" by the observer, and that the more precise the selection has to be, the longer it takes or the more risk there is of error. The times taken may, in absolute terms, be brief, but in most cases they are appreciable and in some are substantial. Evidence is provided by a number of experiments in which times taken to react to stimuli have been found to vary with the degree of selection required. For example, Hilgendorf (1966) required her subjects, when a signal appeared, to move as quickly as possible from a "home" key to make the appropriate response. As soon as they moved, the signal disappeared, so that the time taken before moving could be regarded as a measure of the time required to identify the signal. She found that this time rose linearly with the logarithm of the number of possible signals. The time taken to make the appropriate response also rose in the same manner but much more steeply. Again, in experiments mentioned in Chapter 1, where subjects have been presented with several different signals, such as letters or digits, and been required to react to one only, the time taken to do so has been found to increase with the number of different signals to be ignored (Brebner & Gordon, 1962, 1964). Reaction times in similar tasks have also been found to rise when the number of different signals to which a response has to be made has been increased beyond one, even though the same response is made to all of them (Nickerson & Feehrer, 1964).

Two further relevant lines of evidence may be noted. One is from experiments on *scanning*. In these experiments, the subject scans through a list of, say, letters or words and notes the presence or absence of particular items. The time taken for this task has been found to increase with the number of different possible items in the list (Oostlander & de Swart, 1966; Gordon, 1968), with the number of different items being sought in any one scan (Kaplan & Carvellas, 1965; Kaplan et al., 1966; Nickerson, 1966), and when the definition of a class of words or other items sought is wide rather than narrow (Foster, 1962; Neisser & Beller, 1965).

Second, experiments have shown that the time taken to classify objects rises with the number of criteria of classification. Thus, for example, Nickerson (1967) found it took longer to identify shapes as red *or* circular, or as red *and* circular, than either as red or as circular alone. Identifying in terms of three criteria—say, red, circular, and large—took longer still.

Although the time taken for selection often seems to rise linearly with the logarithm of the number of alternatives, it does not always do so. In these cases the time taken seems to depend on the *discriminability* of the items to be selected from those to be rejected or ignored. Thus, for example, Neisser (1963) found that scanning for the letter Q among other rounded letters was slower than scanning for it among angular letters. It can perhaps be argued that this is the basis of the more general relationship—the larger the set from which items are to be chosen, the greater the likelihood of poor discriminability. If so, both are examples of the principle that time taken for identification depends on how precisely the item has to be observed, or in other words, how much detail has to be noted in it.

According to this principle, we should expect greater accuracy if attention can be concentrated on one part of a figure than if it has to be spread over the whole figure. Attneave (1957) found this to be so in an experiment in which subjects had to associate names with sets of irregular polygons. Each set of polygons was constructed by making minor variations in a basic design. He found that learning was better when all the variations were made to the same corner rather than to different corners of the figures.

The full benefits of such partial inspection may, however, not always

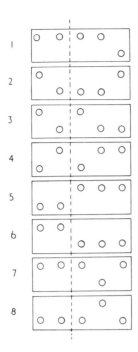

Figure 3.1. *Patterns used by Bricker.*

be realized, because subjects seem to find it difficult to ignore parts of a display even though they are not necessary for correct identification. For instance, Bricker (1955) found that identification of the patterns shown in Figure 3.1 was quicker when the two items on the left of each arrangement were omitted, than when all five were shown. Such findings raise the interesting question of why, if selecting part of the display and excluding the rest would have made identification easier, did subjects not do this? It suggests that the cost of making the selection in terms of time, effort, or possibility of error may sometimes more than offset the extra "work" involved in attending to redundant parts of the display.

The mechanism of selection

There is growing neurological evidence that the various features of the stimuli that impinge upon the organism are sorted out by a complex system of analyzers at various levels in the sense organs and perceptual centers in the brain. The system of analyzers, or as we shall for convenience call it, "the analyzer," is in many ways analogous to a set of resonant electronic tuned filters, although the analogy cannot be pressed very far because many of the neural mechanisms which are known to underlie the simpler stages of analysis are of a different nature.

The most elementary analysis of stimulation is by the various sense organs, with the eye reacting to light, the ear to sound waves, and so on. Further stages of analysis occur within the several sense organs, for example, of wavelength (subjectively color) and intensity of light in the eye, and of frequency (subjectively pitch) and intensity of sound in the ear. More complex analysis occurs in the brain. This has been shown especially for the visual cortex, where analysis is made of lines, angles, movement, verticality, and horizontality (Hubel & Wiesel, 1962, 1968). It has also been argued that the microscopic anatomy of the visual cortex suggests that it carries out a type of Fourier analysis of incoming stimuli in a way which could account both for the perception of more elaborate patterns, and for their recognition, irrespective of their position on the retina (Kabrisky, 1966; Kabrisky et al., 1970). It seems reasonable to suppose that still more complex analyses are to be accounted for in terms of similar types of mechanisms.

Throughout, we can see the important principle that the identification of particular features of a stimulus is associated with the state of particular cells or groups of cells. From this it is only a short conceptual step to the idea that all categories of identification—that is, all the different patterns or objects it is possible to identify—are represented by the states of particular groups or patterns of cells, and that an incoming stimulus is identified according to the group or pattern it affects most (Treisman, 1960). Such identification takes a brief but appreciable time—at least a few milliseconds—and we may conceive of the state of the particular cells as gradually building up over a period of time so that some become more active, or potentially active, than others.

Sources of bias in the analyzer

The fact that a person is able to attend selectively to some sources of stimulation, concentrating on them while ignoring others, implies that the analyzer can somehow be biased so that sensitivity to particular features or patterns of stimulation is increased or reduced before stimuli actually arrive. We do not know how this is done, but we can perhaps envisage the process as one in which the potential activity of particular groups of cells is increased or reduced, so that when the stimulus comes its effect is enhanced or partly offset. There seem to be several different sources of such positive and negative bias, which may supplement or counteract each other on particular occasions. Let us consider some of the most important.

1. The processes of adaptation in sense organs and of habituation in more central mechanisms, whereby reactivity to long-continued or regularly repeated stimulation is reduced, can probably be regarded as elementary forms of bias. They seem to operate over widely different time scales. Thus the partial deafness that results from exposure to loud sounds may last for hours, while a visual image held stable at the same point on the retina quickly fades but returns if the image shifts. Such processes of adaptation and habituation indicate that the perceptual system is essentially geared to dealing with changes of stimulation rather than with steady states.

2. A further simple form of bias, operating on a very short time scale, lies

in the interactions between different parts of a sensory field. A good example is the way in which a stimulus at one point on the retina partially inhibits activity in the zone surrounding it, thus enhancing contrast at the edges of patterns and the clarity with which objects stand out from their backgrounds (von Bekesy, 1967).

3. It must be emphasized that, although analysis on any particular occasion may subjectively be concerned with only one sensory mode, data from other senses may also contribute. Thus, it is almost always easier to hear what a person is saying if we can also see the speaker; the effects of seen mouth movements and facial expressions supplement the heard sounds. Again, what is seen at any one moment depends upon a context or conceptual framework which has been built up from visual data supplemented by data from eye-, head-, and body-movements. The framework can be conceived of as a continuing system of biases which provide a context into which each new item of data, whether visual, postural, or otherwise, is received, and to which each new item contributes. We shall consider such frameworks further in a later section of this chapter.

4. Other subtle, complex, and varied biases can be attributed to aftereffects of previous activity in the system. A seemingly straightforward kind of bias is illustrated by the results of experiments in which pictures of objects had to be identified, either when only parts of the outline were present (Verville & Cameron, 1946), or when the pictures were exposed very briefly (Wallace, 1956). Subjects tended to perseverate in the class of identification they chose. Thus, if they had correctly identified one object as, say, a horse, they would identify the next object also as an animal, and, if told this was incorrect, would try other animals before changing to other classes of objects such as vehicles or articles of furniture. Such behavior could be explained by assuming that the activity in the analyzer associated with the animal identified on the first occasion, spread so as to activate the identifications of other animals to some extent, and that this partial activation was still present to a significant extent when the next object was seen.

The concept of bias in a system of this kind provides a powerful means of accounting for the effects of familiarity. The clearest effects are those where a sequence of stimuli leads to a conscious expectation of subsequent items. The standard example of "the mat" being almost inevitably expected after "the cat sat on" will suffice. We may assume that the activity produced by the initial words of the sentence partly activates the subsequent words, so that they are more likely to be identified than others. Consistent with this view is the fact, noted in many studies, that a word which is inappropriate to the sentence in which it occurs may be misheard as a more probable word.

These context effects seem often to depend not only on what has gone before, but also on what follows, implying that the sentence is not heard in a purely sequential manner, but rather as a single whole once it is complete, and that what is then heard depends on the total pattern of biases operating at that moment. If so, it is not difficult to recognize that the effect of learning can be conceived of as the setting up of patterns of bias which come into effect as wholes when certain stimuli impinge upon the senses.

Perseveration and the effects of familiarity can be thought of as due to biases operating respectively on short and long time scales. In the same way, we can identify biases operating on intermediate time scales due, for example, to instructions in a psychological experiment, or to the discrepancies between present state and optimum that we call motives. Thus the classical experiments of Keys et al. (1950) showed that men kept for a substantial period in a state of semistarvation became unusually prone to notice anything to do with food, such as advertisements for foods in magazines.

5. Operating simultaneously with all these sources of bias are random stimuli in the central nervous system. This random activity can be conceived of as adding to, or subtracting from, the bias in various parts of the analyzer to an extent which varies from moment to moment. These internal stimuli may be the source of many errors of performance. For example, the spoken letters b, c, d, e, g, p, t, and v tend to be confused. The common vowel sound they share would mean that each would partially activate the rest. Such partial activation, combined with the effects of random activity, might easily result in the overall activation of the letter actually presented being less than that of another letter causing, say, b, to be identified as d.

The combination of random neural activity with various sources of bias provides a much more general explanation of many everyday slips of the tongue and other momentary confusions than does the Freudian view that they are due to the intrusion of repressed desires (Freud, 1914). For example, I remember saying on one occasion while walking along a street, "I wonder whether X will sell his car?" when I should have said, "I wonder whether X will sell his house?" We had just passed a garage, and it was clear in retrospect that doing so had produced a bias towards cars which could easily, when combined with momentary random neural activity, have caused the word "car" to be substituted for "house."

In general, what we have said so far indicates that present sensory data are automatically analyzed in terms of an organization which combines the effects of inherent constitution of the organism, long-term learning, and the immediately preceding situation. Various parts of the analyzer become more and more differentiated with time, as signals from the sense organs continue to impinge upon it. We can think of it as eventually reaching a critical state in which some part of it fires, and so triggers the next link in the chain of mechanisms leading from stimulus to response. In subjective terms, a decision is made.

The critical state appears to vary according to needs. For example, if we are crossing the street we will notice that there is a car approaching, but do not usually observe what make or model it is. If, however, we are looking for a friend's car which is to pick us up, we will scrutinize approaching cars in greater detail, to distinguish the one we want. The greater the detail required, the longer it takes to reach a decision. Presumably this means that the decision process itself is subject to bias from preceding conditions and from present needs, aims, and expectations. We may think of these as determining the amount of buildup from external signals needed, and therefore the time required, to fire a correct decision.

The decision may be to take definitive action or to obtain further data. Commonly both functions are involved, although in extreme cases only one or the other may be present. Thus a simple reflex reaction can be regarded as a case where action is taken without further data being sought, while turning the head and eyes towards an object moving in peripheral vision is a case of seeking further data without taking any definitive action.

Simultaneous and successive processing

Analysis of data coming in over different sensory modes must be made simultaneously, rather than successively; otherwise, rapid and close coordination of data from, say, eye and ear would be impossible. There has, however, been considerable controversy as to whether, when a decision has to be made on two or more different features of an item, such as color, shape, and size in Nickerson's (1967) study, these are identified serially or simultaneously. Suppose, for example, a subject has to select from a series of shapes those which are *both* red *and* square. If the conjunctive decisions between red as opposed to other colors and between square as opposed to other shapes are made simultaneously, the overall time taken will roughly equal the time required to decide about color alone or about shape alone, whichever is longer. Because of random variation in the time required to make decisions, the conjunctive decision will tend to take a little longer than this, but probably not much. If the decisions are made successively, the time to decide on both criteria will be the sum of the times required to decide on each criterion alone, in addition to the time required for any purely sensory processes or for the motor action of responding.

Similarly, the time taken by a subject to make the disjunctive decision, about whether a shape is *either* red *or* square, as opposed to neither red nor square, would, if decisions are simultaneous, lie between the times for the longer and shorter of the decisions about color or shape taken singly, since sometimes one and sometimes the other would suffice. If the decisions are successive, the time would sometimes be that for one of the single decisions, sometimes that for the other, and sometimes the sum of both, again in addition to purely sensory or response times.

Nickerson found that, on the whole, his results favored serial identification. The evidence from studies in this area is not entirely clear, and the interpretation of published experiments is often difficult or impossible. Generally speaking, however, the evidence seems to indicate that decisions about different features of an object have, in many cases at least, to be made successively. Perhaps analyses of two or more different criteria are in fact made simultaneously, but the one which reaches a critical state first triggers a decision, and by doing so closes the gate to the translation mechanism for a short time, so that decisions about other criteria are delayed, as outlined in Chapter 1. This would not happen if the critical states were reached almost simultaneously, since a single decision could then incorporate the data from all of them.

Evidence from several studies of scanning using very familiar or highly practiced items suggests simultaneous processing. For example, Neisser (1963) found that when subjects scanned lists of letters for both Q and Z, they took little, if any longer than to scan for whichever was the slower of Q or Z alone. Again, Neisser et al. (1963) found that scanning for ten or five letters took longer than scanning for one initially, but that the times became virtually identical after long practice (see also Corcoran, 1967b).

These latter results have been interpreted to mean that serial processing of different features gives way through practice to simultaneous processing. Other explanations are, however, possible, at least in some cases. For instance, a subject scanning for a large number of letters, may have difficulty initially in remembering which letters are being sought, so that there is improvement with practice due to learning. This, however, can hardly explain Neisser's results when subjects scanned for only two letters. A second possibility is that, in the course of a series of trials, each with different requirements, subjects may improve identification speed in general but find it increasingly difficult to ignore irrelevant data. If this were so, they would, when scanning for single items, inspect more thoroughly than necessary, and a basic successiveness might be masked. A third possibility, especially with a continuous task such as scanning, is that identification of one signal comes to overlap the making of a response to a previous one as portrayed in Figure 1.2. In this case, scanning time may come to be set not so much by the times taken to identify signals, but by the times required to decide whether or not to respond.

There remains the possibility that, in the course of practice, the method of identification does not change from successive to simultaneous, but from analysis in terms of individual features to a process of matching the incoming data against a set of complex patterns specific to the task or long ingrained in the subject's experience. An explanation along these lines would link perceptual selection to many facts of perceptual integration, memory, habit formation, and problem solving, which seem to depend on imposing preformed "templates" or "schemata" onto incoming data. We shall consider these processes in the next section.

Perceptual integration

Turning from selection to integration, two approaches seem especially important. One is the view that perceptual analysis attempts to minimize the number
of items required to account for data adequately. For example, Hochberg
and McAlister (1953), who showed subjects designs similar to those in Figure
3.2, suggested that A and B should be seen as three-dimensional more than
C and D because the number of lines and angles required to specify A and
B in two dimensions is greater than that required for C and D. Thus, for
specification in two dimensions, A and B each require 16 lines and 26 angles,
whereas C requires 13 lines and 20 angles and D 12 lines and 18 angles.
In three dimensions all patterns require 12 lines and 24 angles. These researchers
indeed found that the percentage of three-dimensional responses followed
expectation in being 98.7, 99.3, 51.0, and 40.0 for A, B, C, and D respectively.
A, B, and D were therefore most often seen in the more economical way
while C, which required about the same number of elements in either
specification, was seen about equally often in each way.

The second approach assumes that ease of perception depends on the
extent to which one part of a pattern can be inferred from another. It is
well illustrated by a "guessing game" (based on Attneave, 1954) used for

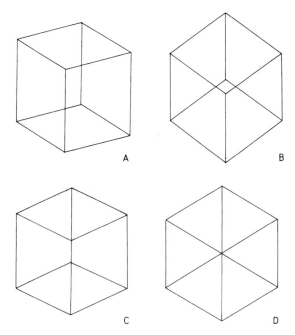

Figure 3.2. *Four projections of a cube.*

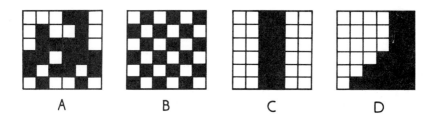

Figure 3.3. *Designs used in a "guessing game." The subject is required to guess, without seeing the design, whether each square is black or white, beginning at the top left-hand corner and proceeding from left to right along each row in turn.*

some years in class experiments at the Cambridge University Psychological Laboratory. The experimenter has a grid containing a pattern of the type shown in Figure 3.3. The subject cannot see the experimenter's grid, but has his or her own blank grid, and is required to guess whether each square in turn will be white or black. The experimenter tells the subject the correct answer after each guess, and the subject records it on the grid, thus gradually building up a copy of the experimenter's grid. If the pattern is random, as in Figure 3.3A, the subject, on the average, cannot guess better than 50 percent correct. If, however, the pattern is not random, as in Figure 3.3B and C, the subject can quickly detect the regularities and thereafter makes no more errors. If the pattern changes, as in Figure 3.3D, the subject makes a few errors around the point of change, but none once its nature and direction have been recognized. It is not suggested that anyone does in fact scan a pattern like this in the course of ordinary perception, but the game serves to emphasize that, once regularities have been detected, much of the rest of the pattern can be inferred.

Both these approaches, especially the second, imply that some sort of *constants* are extracted from the data presented, and that items not included in these constants have to be noted, or specified, separately. Both also imply that, insofar as language reflects experience, the ease of specifying a pattern verbally and the number of words or phrases required, gives an approximate measure of the readiness with which it will be perceived.

Applications of these approaches have recently been made to classical principles of perception. For example, objects tend to be seen as grouped when they are similar in shape, or close together or continue along a line; and simple, regular, or symmetrical patterns are usually easier to perceive than those which are complex or irregular (Simon, 1967; Welford, 1968; Glanzer et al., 1968). We shall not try to survey these applications, but will confine our discussion to some seemingly important implications and extensions of these two approaches to perceptual integration.

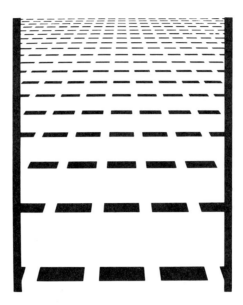

Figure 3.4. *Perspective gradient used by Vickers.*

Extraction of gradients

A considerable advance in understanding the perception of three-dimensional space was made by Gibson (1950) regarding the nature of perspective effects. Perspective, he suggested, results from extracting a rate of change or *gradient* of size from similar objects at different distances in space. Such objects, although they subtend different visual angles, become in an important sense *invariant* once the gradient has been recognized. Perception may, in this way, be regarded as tending to maximize the invariance in the data presented. An example of a perspective gradient is shown in Figure 3.4. If the pattern is regarded as two-dimensional and perpendicular to the line of sight, all the black broken lines and the spaces between them are of different sizes or shapes. Once a gradient has been extracted, all become similar although at different apparent distances.

The gradient appears to be extracted at some cost. Vickers (1971) has shown that if Figure 3.4 is covered by a card except for the bottom two rows of bars, these rows are not likely to be seen as three-dimensional. If the card is slowly raised to expose further rows, the three-dimensional effect suddenly appears. The same is true for Figure 3.5, but the changeover from two to three dimensions comes later. It seems reasonable to suppose that this is so because the amount of data per row rendered invariant is greater in Figure 3.4 than in Figure 3.5. In the former figure, length, width, shape, and distances between bars all become invariant; in the latter, only distances.

We seem to have here an example of an economy principle: the gradient is extracted when the amount of data rendered invariant is enough to offset the cost of extraction. What is meant by "cost" in this context has yet to be determined, although it can be defined operationally in terms of the gain in invariance required to offset it. Evidence confirming the general line of argument comes from the greater ease and accuracy with which objects are located in space as the number of surrounding objects from which a gradient can be extracted increases.

The gradients in Figures 3.4 and 3.5 are for flat surfaces. Gibson emphasized that these are not the only ones that can be extracted; different gradients give impressions of curved surfaces, either concave or convex, and the *rate* of change affects the apparent angle of slope relative to the observer's line of regard. Nor are such gradients confined to spatial arrangements. The fact, for example, that objects retain the same apparent whiteness when seen in different illuminations, appears to be due essentially to the same principle. It is not generally realized that perception of white and black has little to do with the absolute amounts of light reflected by objects. A few readings with a photometer, or looking at objects through a narrow tube which excludes sight of their surroundings, will reveal that a black object in good light—say, near a window—may be reflecting substantially more light than a white object in shadow further into the room. The fact that one looks black and the other white implies that the observer has extracted, albeit unconsciously, a gradient of brightness, and has thus rendered the relation between black and white invariant in the different illuminations.

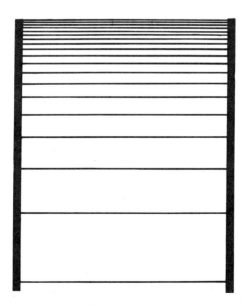

Figure 3.5. *A simplified perspective gradient used by Vickers.*

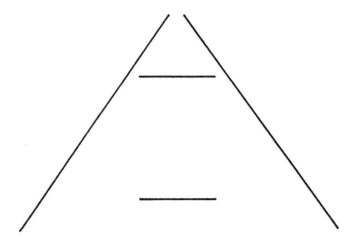

Figure 3.6. *A version of the Ponzo illusion. The two horizontal lines are the same length.*

Once a gradient has been extracted, all objects within its field tend to be scaled accordingly. This has been held to account for many of the geometrical illusions, such as that of Figure 3.6, in which the lower horizontal line tends to look shorter than the upper; it is assumed that the observer automatically treats the converging lines as a perspective gradient and that the horizontal lines are scaled in terms of this gradient (Gregory, 1966).

Perspective gradients may not be entirely accurate in scaling objects. It has, for example, been known since the pioneer work of Thouless (1931) that if, say, a circular disc is seen as tilted, an observer asked to assess the elliptical shape it projects to the eye will judge it to be fatter than it really is. Similar effects occur with other judgments: for instance, the projections of distant objects are judged too large, and horizontal distances are judged as shorter and shorter as they become more distant (Gilinsky, 1951). In sum, these distortions make the visual scene appear foreshortened and tilted up, as though viewed a little more from above than it really is. We can only speculate upon the origins of such a system; it may possibly have some biological utility in enabling the distant scene to be examined, in a sense, more closely.

Transformations over time

As an observer moves, the relative positions of objects at different distances in the field of vision also change, and slightly different views of the objects themselves are obtained. Gibson stressed that these changes of position and view form gradients in terms of which the *stability* of positions in space, and the shapes of solid objects, are recognized. The particular positions and shapes perceived are those which are invariant under the coordinated set of changes and transformations produced by the observer's movement. In the same way, departure from such invariance is an indication that the objects themselves are moving or changing shape (Gibson, 1968).

It seems possible also that the *potential* effects of change of position may influence the perception of some static objects. For example, if minor perspective effects are neglected, all four patterns in Figure 3.2 are projections of a cube, but they are not all equally probable. A real outline cube would only be seen as D by an observer who viewed it with one eye from a fixed position. Viewing with one eye would also be necessary for C, and movement would be permissible only along a vertical axis. The latter condition, although not the former, would still apply to B. These limitations would not apply to A: the size of the small parallelogram in the middle would differ according to precise orientation, but the same general pattern would remain with both vertical and horizontal movement and whether viewed with one eye or two.

We thus see that incoming data are treated in both spatial and temporal terms which usually seem to operate together. Both spatial and temporal characteristics occur in several different orders of magnitude. For example, when we look at a picture, we may be aware of certain details of brushwork or the depicting of particular objects, and at the same time we may note broad features of overall composition and design. Similarly, when we read a book, we are concerned not only with the meanings of individual words or sentences but with the content of paragraphs and chapters, and often with broader characteristics such as the style of writing. It is, perhaps, not too farfetched to suggest that a person makes a kind of Fourier analysis of incoming data, treating their characteristics in terms of varying time scales or degrees of generality.* If so, the identification of characteristic time scales required or used seems to be a promising method of analyzing the demands of tasks, of specifying methods of training perceptual performance, and of defining certain facets of individual ability and personality.

Effects of familiarity

The effects discussed so far have had little, if anything, to do with familiarity, and are therefore matters of basic capacity rather than skill. We have already mentioned that if objects are inspected through a narrow tube which excludes sight of their surroundings, a black object in good light may be seen as brighter than, and look whiter than, a white object in shadow. Viewing them in this way does not, however, affect the perception of one as black and the other as white when they are again viewed in the context of other objects. In the same way, the horizontal lines in Figure 3.6 look different in length even though we know they are the same. Again, we extract gradients from data not because we are used to seeing them in this way, but because doing so increases invariance.

It is, indeed, possible to perceive something in an unfamiliar way if

---

*This type of Fourier analysis is of a different order of magnitude from that discussed by Kabrisky et al., 1970.

the invariance is thereby made greater. For example, the now famous Ames distorted rooms are often assumed to look rectangular because we are used to seeing rectangular rooms, but the reason seems rather to be that they are so scaled that their projection at the eye has maximum invariance when they are seen as rectangular. A rectangular room can be made to look distorted by suitable scaling of windows, wall-panels, and floorboards so as to give maximum invariance when it is seen as other than rectangular.

On the other hand, much of the ordering of perceptual data in real-life situations undoubtedly depends upon the application of patterns or "templates," or as Bartlett (1932) termed them, "schemata," built up in the course of experience. The imposition of such a schema enables complex data to be apprehended as a unitary whole, and seems to increase the discriminability of a pattern from irrelevant background "noise" (Thierman, 1968). Typically the fit does not have to be precise, and the schema itself constantly seems to be modified by further experience. For example, the category "modern car" includes a range of shapes, sizes, and makes which change substantially during a lifetime. Bartlett noted that complex line drawings that could be matched to a familiar object were regarded as "simpler" by subjects than less objectively complex drawings that could not be readily linked to familiar objects. Similarly, Erdmann and Neal (1968) found familiar words to be about as legible as single letters, although unfamiliar words were less so.

Bartlett indicated that the choice of schemata used was influenced by social conventions and the observer's individual interests. The possibility of deliberately shaping perception by introducing bias towards particular schemata was illustrated in the classical experiment of Carmichael et al. (1932) who showed, for example, that the reproduction of two circles, joined by a short line and exposed briefly, differed according to whether the observer was told beforehand that he was going to see a pair of spectacles or a dumbbell. This result indicates what has been repeatedly demonstrated, that when a schema is applied, detail which is apparently observed is often in fact inferred; details brought by the schema seem to be incorporated into the resulting perception. Details in the stimulus which do not fit in the schema are either ignored or become what Bartlett termed "dominant details" which are specially noticed. Those details ignored do not seem to be completely lost, since they can in some circumstances be reported if the observer is challenged to do so (Earhard, 1968).

Thus, the observer seems to apply some familiar category to incoming data. If the category adequately fits the data, perception of deviant details is at least partially suppressed. If, however, the lack of fit is substantial in one or two respects, the deviant features are specified separately. Attneave (1954) has argued that such a procedure could still be much more economical than no categorization. We might add that it could often be more economical to accept a *quickly found* schema and to specify deviant details, than to make an extensive search of the material stored in memory for a more precise category.

On the practical side, the building and applying of templates or schemata seem to be of importance in relation to industrial inspection (Thomas, 1962). Observation of inspectors at work reveals that they often do their work much faster than classical studies of the time needed for discrimination and choice would lead us to expect. Most spectacular is, perhaps, the inspection of printed sheets, which an inspector may flip through rapidly, and yet readily note where some fault in the printing has occurred.

Laboratory studies have shown that in many cases *identity* can be recognized relatively quickly (Sekuler & Abrams, 1968). We should, therefore, expect that an inspector would benefit from building up a schema of a perfect article to apply to each example as it came along, rejecting deviations from it. In the most rapid inspection tasks, the succession of perfect articles might take on the character of a continuous single pattern which changes when a fault occurs. The development of a schema might, however, sometimes lead to difficulties. If it were too precise and detailed, the deviations observed would sometimes be within tolerable limits so that satisfactory articles would be rejected. If this happened, the inspector would have to make a more complex judgment of whether an article was *similar* to a standard within a permitted range of variation. This type of judgment was shown by Sekuler and Abrams to take considerably longer than recognition of identity.

Building perceptual frameworks

Gibson emphasized that when we perceive an object of substantial size, we do not see all the relevant details at a single glance: our eyes rove over it, observing first one part, then another. Our total perception is thus not the same as the observation in any one glance: rather it is a *construct* built by integrating together the data from many different glances. Such integration seems to be readily achieved when all the data are present together, so that the data in focal attention in one glance are those more peripherally observed in others. When all data are not present at once, integration may still be achieved provided they arrive within a fairly short period of time. Experiments in which parts of patterns have been shown sequentially have indicated that the accuracy of integration falls rapidly with increasing times between the exposures of the different parts: for example, from 0 to 100 msec (Eriksen & Collins, 1968), or from 125 to 800 msec (Garner & Gottwald, 1968). The former range of times is similar to that noted in Chapter 1 during which successive data could be passed together from the perceptual mechanism to the translation mechanism before the "gate" between them closed. Garner and Gottwald suggest that integration achieved at longer intervals is not truly perceptual, in that the pattern is never perceived all at once as a whole. The integration is rather a matter of recognizing that the various parts would form a unitary pattern if they were shown all together.

Once integration has been achieved, it seems as if an enduring, stable framework has been built up which is immediately available as a whole. It is these visual frameworks that constitute what Gibson called our "visual world," in terms of which we maintain orientation. They provide a context to which fresh incoming data are either congruent and readily incorporated, or deviant, in which case attention is concentrated on them and further analysis is carried out. In the same way, these frameworks lead to the stimulating idea that perception can be conceived of as a running hypothesis, by which events at any one moment are compared with expectations brought from the immediate past. Such a concept is consistent with the idea of perception as economical, in the sense that attention is concentrated at temporal points of change, just as we saw it was at spatial points of change in Attneave's guessing game (Figure 3.3).

The conditions which favor the building and maintenance of these frameworks are not fully understood, but the experiments on integration that we have already noted suggest that they depend to a considerable extent on some form of short-term retention, presumably in the short-term store shown in Figure 1.1. Additional evidence that this is so can perhaps be seen in the loss of orientation often shown by patients suffering from impaired short-term memory. Some further understanding might be gained from studies of the estimation of averages (Spencer, 1961, 1963; Anderson, 1968). These studies have shown, for instance, that the span of data that can be judged is limited, and that highly deviant data tend to be overweighted. The task of understanding the nature of perceptual frameworks is, however, a challenging one in which several different parameters seem to be emerging. Some of the most potentially promising leads are coming from the study of complex process operations in industry. The skilled operator appears to build a conceptual framework or "model" of the process he is using and of its manner of functioning. The model is sometimes crude, even bizarre, but may still nevertheless be highly effective (Crossman, 1960; Beishon, 1967).

Summary

Perceptual coding involves processes of selection and integration of incoming data. Both selection and integration lessen the number of discrete units or items about which decisions have to be made.

Selection is made in part on the basis of sources of data, in part on sensory qualities, and in part on semantic grounds. Selection seems to be carried out by an analyzing mechanism analogous to a filter which appears to be biased for or against particular classes of material. These biases may result from sensory adaptation and interaction, the aftereffects of previous activity, familiarity, expectations, aims, and desires. The analyzer is affected by random neural activity which interacts with various biases to produce errors. There is some controversy about whether analysis of different features of stimuli is simultaneous or successive; almost certainly both types occur.

Recent approaches to integration in the perception of objects stress the roles of economy of specification and the inference of one part of a design from another. Perception seems to be a process which maximizes invariance in the objects perceived, both in space and time. In many cases, such as in space perception and the constancy of shape, size, and whiteness, this occurs automatically and is little if at all affected by knowledge and familiarity. Probably most everyday perceptual integration depends, however, on the application of familiar "schemata" or "templates" to incoming data. These schemata tend to shape perception by adding to the percept details in the familiar schema which are not in the actual data. Details in the data which do not fit with the schemata are either ignored or specified separately. The amount of detail specified appears to vary according to the degree of precision required in the situation.

The effect of the whole process of selection and integration is to build up perceptual frameworks with both spatial and temporal dimensions, into which incoming data are fitted, and which in their temporal aspect make perception a kind of running hypothesis which each incoming datum confirms or modifies.

Choice of response

4

As we saw in Chapter 1, reaction time contains contributions from the three main stages shown in Figure 1.1, and the total time taken to react depends on the times required by all three stages. In Chapter 2, we discussed a case in which choice of response was held constant while perceptual difficulty was varied by making the signals difficult to distinguish from one another. In this chapter, we shall consider cases in which perceptual difficulty is minimized by making signals clearly distinct, but where the number of alternative responses and their relationships to the signals are varied.

In most of the cases we shall consider, a different signal corresponds to each response, so that the subject must identify a signal as well as choose a response. As we noted in Chapter 3, the times required for both identification and choice rise with the number of alternative signals and responses concerned. Both of these times seem to follow similar lawful relationships with the number of alternatives, and models to account for choice reaction time have seldom tried to distinguish between them. Identification tends, however, to be a much smaller component of the total time than choice of response, so that these models can reasonably be assumed to deal mainly with the times required for choice of response in the translation mechanism.

Hick's information theory law

An important insight into the problem of why reaction time rises with degree of choice was made by Hick (1952a), who proposed that, when making choices, subjects resolve uncertainty or gain "information" at a constant rate. Hick based his view on the analysis of two sets of experimental data, his own and those of Merkel (1885). In these experiments there were, in different trials, from 1 to 10 alternative signals, each responded to by pressing a different key. Hick found that if the number of possible signals is taken as n and reaction time is plotted against log $(n + 1)$, the observed reaction times for different numbers of signals lie on a straight line which also passes through the origin, as shown in Figure 4.1. We can thus write

$$\text{Mean choice reaction time} = K \log (n + 1) \qquad (4.1)$$

where K is a constant. If we work in logarithms to the base 2, $\log_2 (n + 1) = 1$ when $n = 1$, so that K is the simple reaction time. The $\log_2$ unit is known in information theory as the *bit*, and can be thought of as a choice between two equally likely alternatives or as the halving of an initial uncertainty. It has proved a convenient unit for describing and comparing a wide range of experimental conditions and performances, without having any truly explanatory value.

The obvious question arises, why $(n + 1)$ and not n? Hick pointed out that if a subject is uncertain when a signal will appear, he must decide, when it does appear, not only which signal it is, but also whether a signal has occurred at all. Failure to make these two decisions results either in reaction when there is no signal present or failure to react when there is one. The additional task of guarding against such errors can be conceived of as adding one to the number of possible conditions to be distinguished—instead of dealing with signals 1, 2, 3, ...n, the subject must deal with states

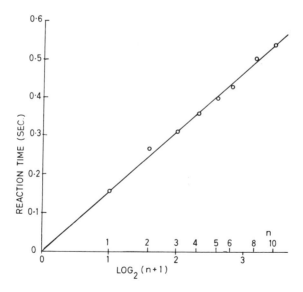

Figure 4.1. *Data from a choice-reaction experiment by Hick plotted in terms of Equation 4.1.*

corresponding to 0, 1, 2, 3, ...*n*. We may denote the sum of the possibilities including *No Signal* as *N*, defining *N* as the equivalent total number of equally probable alternatives from which the subject has to choose, and may then rewrite Equation 4.1 as

$$\text{Mean choice reaction time} = K \log N \qquad (4.2)$$

This formulation has become known as *Hick's law*. It should be understood that this is an "ideal" formula and that time lags in the apparatus or in the making of a response may add a constant to the time.

Hick's line of approach is supported by three further findings:

(a) The amount of information transmitted in a choice reaction task is reduced if the signals are not all of equal frequency. The amount of information due to uncertainty about which signal will occur can be worked out by summing the amounts of information conveyed by each signal weighted according to the probability of its occurrence. We can therefore write in place of log *N* in Equation 4.2

$$\sum_{i=0}^{n} p_i \log \left(\frac{1}{p_i} \right) \qquad (4.3)$$

where p_i is the probability of each possibility in the set taken in turn. This expression reduces to log *N* when all the probabilities are equal. Unequal probabilities reduce the amount of uncertainty and thus the magnitude of expression 4.3, and have been found to produce correspondingly shorter reaction times (Hyman, 1953).

(b) Information transmitted is also reduced when signals tend to follow one another in recognizable sequences or when any signal is followed by any other more often than expected by chance, even though the overall signal frequencies are equal. This is really an extension of the foregoing case. The probabilities of different signals are functions of previous signals, and are thus unequal at any given point in the series, although the inequalities even out over the series as a whole. Hyman found the expected shortening of average reaction times in these cases also.

(c) The amount of information gained is reduced if the subject makes errors. The amount gained when errors are present is given by the equation

$$\text{Information gained} = \sum p_s \log \left(\frac{1}{p_s} \right) + \sum p_r \log \left(\frac{1}{p_r} \right) \qquad (4.4)$$

$$- \sum p_{sr} \log \left(\frac{1}{p_{sr}} \right)$$

where p_s is the probability of each signal, p_r the probability of each response and p_{sr} the probability of each signal-response pair. When there are no errors, so that each signal always leads to its corresponding response, Equation 4.4 reduces to Equation 4.3.

Hick found that the shortening of reaction times when substantial numbers of errors were made was by approximately the amounts expected. Howell and Kreidler (1963) and Fitts (1966), who compared groups of subjects performing choice reaction tasks with instructions for speed, for accuracy, or for both, confirmed that overall rates of information gain were not significantly different for the three types of instruction, although the balance between speed and accuracy was shifted as the instructions required.

Equation 4.4 provides a means of combining speed and accuracy into a single score, and emphasizes the important fact that times for different tasks are comparable only if errors are held constant. Conversely, error rates can be compared only if times are held constant.

Guarding against false reactions

The $+1$ in Hick's formulation has not always proved easy to understand, and an alternative equation proposed by Hyman (1953) has often been preferred. He proposed in place of Equation 4.1

$$\text{Choice reaction time} = a + b \log n \tag{4.5}$$

where a is the simple reaction time and $b \log n$ represents the increase over the simple reaction time due to the need for identification and choice.

On the whole, Equation 4.1 fits the facts better than Equation 4.5, but often there is little to choose between them and in some cases Equation 4.5 provides the better fit. The reason for the variability is indicated in a reformulation of the problem by Smith (1976). He argued that a subject has to build up a central state in favor of a particular response as opposed to others to a criterion level, and that a response is made when this level is reached. The approach is analogous to Vickers' accumulator model outlined in Chapter 2. Smith assumed that

$$\text{Reaction time} = K \log \left(n \frac{C}{E} + 1 \right) \tag{4.6}$$

where E is the strength of the incoming signal in terms of signal-to-noise ratio, and C is a measure of the criterion level at which a response is initiated. C is low in conditions stressing speed rather than accuracy, and becomes higher as the requirement for accuracy rises. When $C = E$, Equation 4.6 is equivalent to Hick's Equation 4.1. The effect when C exceeds E can be seen if Equation 4.6 is rewritten

$$\text{Reaction time} = K \left[\log \left(n + \frac{E}{C} \right) + \log C - \log E \right] \tag{4.7}$$

As C becomes large or E small, the fraction E/C approaches zero. At the same time ($\log C - \log E$) introduces a constant increase regardless of n so that, if reaction time is plotted against $\log n$, the intercept is above zero. Equation 4.6 then approximates Hyman's Equation 4.5. It can reasonably be assumed that E was less in Hyman's experiment than in Hick's because the signal lights were less bright. Consistent with this, Hyman's reaction times were somewhat longer than Hick's for each degree of choice.

Further application of Hick's law

Hick's law and its extensions seem capable of describing performance in a wide variety of sensory-motor performances. To take only one example, Figure 4.2 shows results obtained by Crossman (1953) for sorting playing cards. The subject held a well-shuffled pack face down in one hand. With the other he turned up the cards one by one and sorted them into various classes as quickly as possible. The number of classes was varied in different trials from 2 up to 26. Additional trials were given in which the cards were in a prearranged order, such as alternate red and black, so as to provide a measure of the time taken to turn and place the cards when no identification or choice was required—in other words, a measure of movement time. The results are shown by the upper line in Figure 4.2. Roughly speaking, time per card is the sum of movement time and $K \log n$, where n is the number of classes. The point that falls farthest away from the line is that for the 13 numbers: these seem often to be easier to deal with than less familiar sets of signals. We shall return to this point later.

We may question whether it is sufficient to estimate movement time

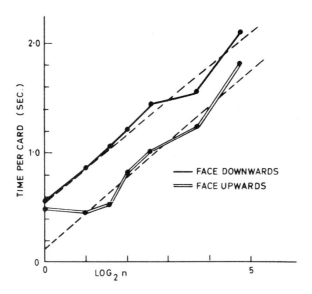

Figure 4.2. *Data from a card-sorting experiment by Crossman. The points along each line represent (from left to right): dealing cards in a prearranged order; sorting into— red/black; pictures/red plain/black plain; suits; red pictures/black pictures/plain in four suits; suits, dividing 6 and below from 7 and above; numbers; numbers, separating red and black.*

by dealing only two piles. Should the cards be dealt into as many piles as there are classes to give a different estimate of movement time for each number of classes? An indication that this elaboration is unnecessary is contained in the results Crossman obtained with the pack held face up so that the subject could see each card immediately after he had removed the previous one. The lower line of Figure 4.2 shows that the time per card was either the movement time or roughly $K \log n$, whichever was the longer. It appears that identification and choice can overlap with movement, so that the two can develop together. Extra movement time required with large numbers of piles can thus be absorbed in the extra time needed for identification and choice.

Models of choice reaction

Theoretical models proposed to account for the logarithmic relationship between reaction time and degree of choice fall into two main groups: serial and simultaneous. *Serial* models assume that subjects make a series of subdecisions, each of which excludes some of the possibilities, until a final identification of one signal and choice of its corresponding response are made. It is usually assumed that each subdecision takes the same amount of time. On this assumption, the simplest serial procedure, that of scanning possible signal sources and their corresponding responses in turn until the one which has occurred is found, would produce results which do not fit the facts. The average number of subdecisions required would be $(n + 1)/2$ so that reaction time would be *linearly* related to the number of possibilities instead of to the *logarithm* of the number.

Two other serial models do, however, yield a logarithmic relationship:

(a) The subject identifies the signal and its corresponding response as lying within one half of the total possibilities, then within one half of this half, and so on. A two-choice task thus requires one decision, a four-choice two decisions, an eight-choice three decisions, and so on (Hick, 1952a). This is the most efficient procedure according to classical information theory (Shannon & Weaver, 1949).

(b) A modification of (a) holds that the subject divides the total possibilities into two, or sometimes three or more classes and inspects each class in turn until the one containing the required signal and response is found. He then subdivides that class and again inspects until he finds the required subclass, and so on (Welford, 1960b, 1968). Thus for each decision between two classes, the subject sometimes requires one inspection and sometimes two—an average of 1.5 if the signals are random and equiprobable.

Similarly, for each decision between three classes a subject sometimes requires one, sometimes two, and sometimes three inspections, resulting in an average of two. The model differs from (a) in assuming that if the required signal and response are not in the class inspected first, the subject does not simply assume that they lie elsewhere, but makes a further inspection or inspections to check positively where they do lie, before proceeding to the next decision.

The *simultaneous* models assume that the subject compares evidence from all the possible signal sources simultaneously, and decides in favor of the response which reaches a criterion value soonest, or for the response which is strongest after a critical time, or as soon as all comparisons have been completed. The process is essentially one of distinguishing the signal and response concerned from random variation in other possible signals and tendencies to response (Hick, 1952b; Christie & Luce, 1956; Rapoport, 1959; Laming, 1966).

The simple serial-dichotomizing model (a) appears to be untenable because it would not allow for a more frequent signal to be responded to faster than a less frequent signal in a two-choice task—one decision would be required in each case. It is also inconsistent with the eight-choice results shown by the heavy line in Figure 4.3. These results were obtained for responses by different fingers to light signals in corresponding positions in a row. Responses by the ring and middle fingers took about 90–100 msec longer than those by the little and index fingers, whereas according to the strict serial-dichotomizing model (a), times for all responses should, on the average, have been the same (Welford, 1971b). These results are also inconsistent with the simultaneous models, which again predict that all responses should, on the average, take the same time.

Both types of models might still be applied to these eight-choice results if it could be shown that either there was some motor factor slowing the responses of the ring and middle fingers, or that the signals corresponding to them were less discriminable. A motor factor seems to be excluded on two grounds. First, the differences in reaction time by the different fingers were reduced or absent in the four- and two-choice results also shown in Figure 4.3. Second, when the lights corresponding to the little and ring and to the middle and index fingers were reversed, reactions by the little fingers, which were formerly the fastest, became the slowest, as shown in the upper line of Figure 4.3.

Differences in the discriminability of the light positions are also an unlikely explanation, because Alegria and Bertelson (1970) found the ring and middle fingers were still slower than the others when the signals were digits all shown in one position. Such difficulty of discrimination as existed seemed to be between adjacent *keys* rather than signals: virtually all errors were due to pressing the key next to the one which was correct. This presumably means that the buildup in the motor cortex which leads to the depression of a particular finger spreads to some extent to the cortical areas of other

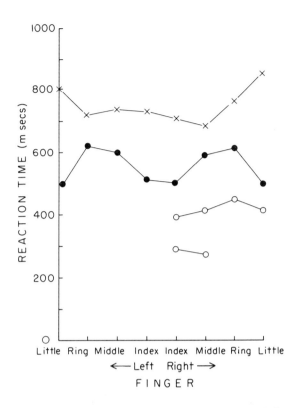

Figure 4.3. *Mean reaction times recorded in eight-, four-, and two-choice tasks (Welford, 1971). The relationships between the positions of the signal lights and response keys were direct except in the case shown in the top line. Here pairs of lights were reversed so that the one at the extreme left of the row was responded to by the left ring finger, the next by the left little finger, and so on.*

fingers. However, it seems unlikely that this can explain the differences between the fingers shown in Figure 4.3. Reaction time to a particular signal can be greatly shortened if the subject is instructed in advance to attend especially to it and to its corresponding response. This is shown on Figure 4.4. If this meant that the buildup for that finger was to some extent made in advance, or that the criterion for responding was lowered, we should expect a relatively high proportion of errors due to this response being given in place of adjacent ones. No such bias was found, so a different explanation must be sought.

The results shown in Figures 4.3 and 4.4 are satisfactorily accounted for by the alternative serial model (b), and the results obtained when concentrating on one of two alternatives in a two-choice task provide a means of testing it quantitatively. In a two-choice task, we may suppose that one inspection is needed to identify the signal and response on which attention is concentrated, and a second to identify the other signal and response. The

Models of choice reaction **63**

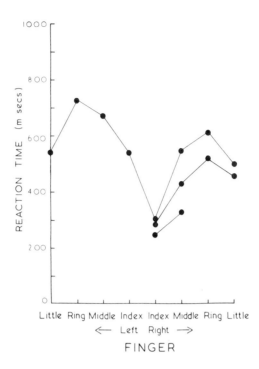

Figure 4.4 *Mean reaction times in eight-, four-, and two-choice tasks, showing the effects of concentrating attention on the responses by the right index finger and its corresponding light (Welford, 1971).*

difference between the average reaction times for the attended and unattended alternatives should therefore be one inspection time. Mean inspection times obtained in this way for different groups of subjects have been about 80–100 msec (Welford, 1971b, 1975). These figures are not very different from those obtained by Vickers et al. (1972) and Nettelbeck (1973a) mentioned in Chapter 2, and it is tempting to regard the two measures as being of fundamentally the same functional unit.

A dichotomizing decision, such as that between the index and middle fingers in the two-choice task of Figure 4.3, will require, as mentioned previously, an average of 1.5 inspection times since the correct signal and response will be reached on half the trials in one inspection, and on half in two. We can, therefore, think of a two-choice reaction time as being made up of two components: 1.5 inspection times, and a "basic time" which includes the time required to observe that a signal has occurred together with any time taken by purely sensory and motor processes and mechanical delays in the apparatus. We should expect the mean four-choice time to be 1.5 inspection times longer than the mean two-choice, and the mean eight-choice to be 1.5 inspection times longer still. This is illustrated in the results shown in Figure 4.3 and in lines A and B of Table 4.1.

Table 4.1. *Observed and predicted mean reaction times (in msec) with different strategies of search.*

Lights and keys	Observed reaction time and 95% confidence limits	Predicted reaction time	Strategy postulated
A 0000	415 ± 7	418	2 × 2
B 00000000	553 ± 8	556	2 × 2 × 2
C 0000*0000*	516 ± 8	510	4 × 2
D .000000.	478 ± 8	478	3 × 2
E . .000000	477 ± 7	478	3 × 2
F 00.00.00	443 ± 7	445)	3 × 2 with
		)	last group
G 0.0000.0	443 ± 7	445)	inspected
		)	serially
H 000. .000	521 ± 9	522	2 × 2 × (2 or 1)

A, B, AND C WERE OBTAINED FROM A GROUP OF THREE SUBJECTS WITH AN AVERAGE INSPECTION TIME OF 92 MSEC AND A BASIC TIME OF 142 MSEC (WELFORD, 1971b, 1973). D, E, F, G, H WERE OBTAINED FROM A GROUP OF FIVE SUBJECTS WITH AN AVERAGE INSPECTION TIME OF 100 MSEC AND A BASIC TIME OF 128 MSEC (WELFORD, 1975).

We can account for the reaction times to the lights corresponding to the little and index fingers being shorter than those to the ring and middle fingers by assuming that the subject tends to inspect the former before the latter. Why this should be so is another matter, but it is probably connected with the tendency of the perceptual system to concentrate on boundaries.

If the alternative serial model (b) is correct, or approximately so, it follows that the effects of imbalance in the frequencies of different signals will follow not the "information" each transmits, but the number of inspections needed to distinguish them. In particular, for accurate performance of a two-choice task, the maximum mean difference between the reaction times to the more and less frequent signals will be one inspection time. Hyman (1953) noted that the reaction times to more and less frequent signals were closer together than a strict information analysis would predict, and in fact no studies appear to have found that mean differences of reaction time to different classes of signal appreciably exceeded 90–100 msec in two-choice tasks with straightforward relationships between signal and response. In most cases the differences have been much less. Differences in reaction time have, of course, been greater with higher degrees of choice or with more complex relationships between signal and response.

In none of the cases has there been any way of estimating inspection time. However, a direct test, using the same subjects as in the experiments of Figures 4.3 and 4.4 in a two-choice task with unbalanced signal frequencies, confirmed that the difference of reaction time to the more and less frequent signals was well within the limits of one inspection time. It was, in fact, close to the difference that would have been expected if subjects had biased their order of inspection in such a way that the proportion of times each signal was inspected first was the same as its probability of occurrence.

Strategies of search

The alternative serial model we have been discussing permits several different strategies of search, some of which are more efficient than others. Choice of strategy seems to depend essentially on two principles. First, it is more efficient to inspect the most likely signal and response or class of signals and responses first. Second, if the total number of possibilities is 3, 4, 5, 6, or 7, dichotomizing is less efficient than simply inspecting the possibilities in turn until the one required is found. With high degrees of choice, an initial division into three or more classes is, therefore, more efficient than division into two classes.

The attainment of efficient strategies seems to be affected by the conditions in an experiment and the layout of the display. Several examples are shown in Table 4.1. Lines A and B show the four- and eight-choice results of Figure 4.3, which are accounted for by strategies of two and three successive dichotomies (2×2 and $2 \times 2 \times 2$) respectively. In the next line, C, results are given by the same subjects with the same eight-choice task, except that they were told to concentrate on the signals and responses of the right hand. Responses by the fingers of the right hand were indeed, on the average, faster than those by fingers of the left hand, while the overall time for all eight fingers was significantly reduced. The subjects appeared to have treated the left hand signals and responses as a four-choice task, inspecting each of two pairs, say, index + middle and ring + little, before passing to the right hand. They would thus have reached the required pair in an average of $(4 + 1)/2$ inspections, i.e., in 2.5 inspections. With an additional average of 1.5 to distinguish the member of the pair concerned, an average total of 4 inspections would have occurred instead of the 4.5 required by a dichotomizing strategy (Welford, 1973). This finding has the interesting practical implication that if initial attention can be concentrated on part of the display, average reaction times may be faster than if attention has to range equally over the whole display. For example, a driver on a main road who knows that all cars on side roads have to yield at intersections will react to events ahead faster than one who must yield to cars approaching from the right.

The remaining lines of Table 4.1 are for six-choice tasks with the same apparatus but without using two of the lights and their corresponding keys (Welford, 1975). Results for D and E, where the signals and responses are all in one block of six, are explained by a strategy involving an initial division into three blocks of two, thus requiring an average of $(3 + 1)/2 = 2, +$ $1.5 = 3.5$ inspections. Results for F and G, where the lights and keys form three separate groups, are explained by a refinement of the same strategy whereby if two groups are inspected without success the third is not taken as a group, but is inspected serially one by one. This last strategy saves, on the average, one inspection on one third of the occasions, so that the overall average becomes 3.17. Detailed examination of the reaction times by different fingers suggests that the possibilities in the six-choice layouts F and G were divided into three groups of two—middle, right, and left—which tended to be inspected in that order.

The last line of Table 4.1, H, shows results where the lights formed two groups of three. Although theoretically this arrangement could be inspected as efficiently as three groups of two, it appears not to have been. The average reaction time was in accordance with the predictions of a progressive dichotomizing strategy. It looks as if the initial division into two determined the pattern for subsequent divisions. This result, taken with the other six-choice results, appears to have some obvious implications for the layout of consoles and instrument panels: items should be in three rather than two groups, with those requiring most immediate action in the middle group, and those requiring least on the left.

Looking back over the results set out in Figures 4.3 and 4.4 and in Table 4.1, it seems clear that with relatively few assumptions about different strategies, the alternative serial classification model (b) enables remarkably accurate predictions of reaction time to be made. It remains to be seen how far the use of efficient strategies can be encouraged by instruction and training.

Errors of choice

We have up to now looked at the process of choice in the translation mechanism mainly from the input end, and considered it as a gradual elimination of possible alternatives until the one which has actually occurred is identified and the response corresponding to it is chosen. First broad classes are eliminated and then narrower ones until the final decision is made. It is instructive to look at the elimination process also from the output end, seeing it as giving rise to a buildup of activity in a small area of the motor cortex to an extent which causes, in the case we have been discussing, one finger to be moved while others remain stationary. We may suppose that excitation produced by the incoming signal is initially spread over all the alternatives, and that each successive stage of elimination concentrates it more and more on one of them, until it reaches the firing level C in Equation 4.6. In this sense, the process is analogous to the focusing of perceptual attention discussed in Chapters 2 and 3.

We have already suggested that there is likely to be some spread of the effect of the buildup in any area to adjacent areas and that this, combined with random noise in the system, provides a plausible reason for the fact that virtually all the errors in the experiments we have been discussing were the result of pressing the key next to the one which was correct. We can further argue that the higher the criterion, the longer the buildup will take, but the fewer the errors that will be made. We can thus understand the tendency for accuracy to fall as speed rises. Pew (1969), who reviewed the results of several studies, showed that the relation between reaction time and accuracy could be represented by the equation

$$\text{Mean reaction time} = a + b \log \frac{\text{(proportion of correct responses)}}{\text{(proportion of errors)}} \quad (4.8)$$

Pew points out that, where there are two alternatives, the log portion of Equation 4.8 is linearly related to the square of d' in the signal detection model. This is consistent with Hick's law, since $(d')^2$ is a linear function of information. Pew's formulation has, however, been challenged by Lappin and Disch (1972a, b) who reviewed various approaches to the problem and found that their own data were better explained by regarding reaction time as linearly related to d' instead of to its square. In either case, the speed-accuracy relationship depends on the magnitude of d' attained when the buildup reaches criterion. It is perhaps worth noting in this connection that in the results shown in Figure 4.3, the average d' between each response and those adjacent to it, as calculated from the errors made, was practically constant at about 4 with all degrees of choice.

The fact that the balance struck between speed and accuracy can be varied by instructions presumably means that it is subject to skill. Pew notes that the effects of practice are to lower both a and b in Equation 4.8. The first suggests that practice either reduces various residual processes which contribute to overall reaction time, or, more probably, lowers the ratio C/E of Equation 4.6. The fall in b implies that practice somehow increases the rate of buildup, probably by producing a closer relationship between perception and choice, as we shall discuss later in this chapter.

Viewing the process of choice as one of a progressive buildup of activity to a critical level in the motor cortex provides an explanation of two further findings not easily accounted for otherwise. First, Seibel (1963) gave subjects a task in which all possible combinations of ten signal lights and response keys were used to yield 1,032 choices. He found that reaction times were very little longer than those obtained in a similar task that used only five lights and keys with one hand to yield 31 choices. We may suppose that the buildup required to strike chords with several fingers at once virtually always distinguishes each finger from its neighbors, and that it does not differ appreciably whether all ten or only the five fingers of one hand are used.

Second, it seems reasonable to suppose that any spread of effect in the motor cortex would affect other areas in proportion to their distance from the focal point, so that errors would be related to the "neural distance" between correct and erroneous responses. There is some evidence from experiments by Blyth (1963, 1964) that this is so. He found that in a four-choice task in which responses were made by the two hands and two feet, the overwhelming majority of errors were due to the substitution of the wrong limb on the correct side. Occasional errors were made with the correct limb on the wrong side, but never with the wrong limb on the wrong side. Further studies by the same experimenter verified that this result did not depend on the layout of the signals but seemed clearly due to responses on the same side being more readily confused than those on opposite sides.

Compatibility, practice, and familiarity

The extent to which reaction time increases with degree of choice differs greatly between one set of conditions and another. Two main factors have been identified: first, what was termed "compatibility" of display and control by Fitts and Seeger (1953)—that is, the directness of the relationships between signals and their corresponding responses—and second, practice and familiarity. We shall consider these in turn.

Compatibility
We may take, as an example, an experiment by Crossman (1956) who investigated the times taken to move from a central position to press particular keys in response to numbered signal lights. Two relationships between signal and response were studied. In one, the more compatible of the two, each signal light was located immediately above its corresponding key; in the other, they were scattered in random positions on a panel. The increase of response time between two and eight choices was much less for the first condition than for the second. Presumably in the first, once the light was identified, the key was also, whereas in the second arrangement, the light had to be identified first and then its number used to locate the corresponding key. In other words, in the second condition the data had to be recoded from digital to spatial form before a response could be chosen, so that the translation mechanism had more "work" to do than when each light was located above its corresponding key. The amount of work is indicated by K in Equations 4.1, 4.2, and 4.6, and by b in Equation 4.5.

Leonard (1959) attempted to produce complete compatibility by using as signals vibrations to the tips of the fingers which were to make the corresponding responses. He found an increase in reaction time from simple to two-choice conditions, but no further rise in four- or eight-choice. Some increase from simple to two-choice conditions is to be expected because, when only one response is required, it can be prepared to an extent that is not possible when two or more responses are called for. Leonard's results, however, can be questioned because he measured reactions from only one finger, which was used in all conditions, and also because he provided more practice with the higher degrees of choice so that effects of compatibility were not clearly distinct from those of practice.

Smith (1976), in repeating Leonard's experiment, avoided these shortcomings. His results, which appear in the top line of Table 4.2, show that between the runs in the eight-choice, the four-choice, and the two-choice conditions, there was a progressive decline in reaction times, although it was small compared with those shown in, say, Figure 4.3. We can see that Smith's results broadly confirm Leonard's in the sense that there is little difference of reaction time between the three degrees of choice. What difference there is might reasonably be attributed to longer time taken for perceptual identification with increase in the number of possible signals. Work by the translation mechanism in both Leonard's and Smith's experiments can be regarded as having been minimal, so that the main increase of reaction time with degree of choice in other experiments is presumably due to the time taken by the translation mechanism to relate signals to responses.

This view is supported when the top line of Table 4.2 is compared with the second and third lines, which set out results for two further conditions studied by Smith. In the "reflected" condition, the stimulus to any finger had to be responded to with the corresponding finger of the other hand, so that the mapping of signals to responses was by mirror-image reflection to positions on the opposite side of the body. In the "shifted" condition, the correct response had to be made by the other hand so that a stimulus to the left little finger was responded to by the right index finger, a stimulus to the left ring finger by the right middle finger, and so on. Both of these conditions obviously involved a more complex relationship between signal and response than the direct condition, and in both, the increase in reaction time with degree of choice was in fact much greater than in the direct condition.

Table 4.2. *Mean reaction times (in msec) to vibratory stimuli delivered to the tips of fingers, with different degrees of compatibility between stimulus and response. Percentages of errors are given in brackets. Data from Smith (1976).*

Relationship between stimulus and response	Runs			Bits per second for rise from 2-choice to 8-choice
	8-choice	4-choice	2-choice	
Direct	246(5.9)	239(5.9)	223(5.4)	87.0
Reflected	628(13.3)	532(9.7)	324(6.9)	6.6
Shifted	858(13.0)	698(9.7)	385(9.7)	4.2

It is clear from the error percentages shown in Table 4.2 that the longer reaction times did not result in greater accuracy.

The translations in these and in the many other studies of compatibility can be divided into two main classes: *symbolic recodings* or *transformations* as studied by Crossman (1956), and *spatial transpositions*, as exemplified in Smith's (1976) experiments.

The question has been raised of how far incompatibility effects in the spatial transformations are due to discrepancies between the spatial layouts of display and control, and how far they arise from the fact that in many cases a stimulus on the right has to be responded to with the left hand and vice versa, so that the stimulus goes to one cerebral hemisphere and the response is made from the other. Appreciable increases of reaction time have been shown when such crossing over is required (e.g., Filbey & Gazzaniga, 1969; Jeeves & Dixon, 1970). However, this is an insufficient explanation, as shown by experiments in which responses were made with the hands crossed. In these experiments, a light on the left has to be responded to by pressing a key on the right with the left hand, so that there is no crossover from one hemisphere to the other. Yet in these cases reaction times are longer than when a light on the left is responded to on the right with the right hand which does require a crossover (Simon et al., 1970; Wallace, 1971; Brebner et al., 1972). It seems as if some lengthening of reaction time results when the spatial relationship is disturbed, either between positions of signal and response, or between positions of hand and response.

As yet there appears to be no way to express the effects of particular transformations or transpositions beyond the rather bald statement that they affect K in Equations 4.1, 4.2, and 4.6, and b in Equation 4.5. Further hypotheses are fragmentary. For example, Kay (1954, 1955; see also Welford, 1958) found that combining both types of translation had a much greater slowing effect on performance than the sum of the effects of each separately; perhaps the translation mechanism is able to handle only one type of translation at a time. Again, Griew (1958) found that the increase of reaction time with degree of choice when lights and keys were well separated was about double that when the lights were positioned immediately above their corresponding keys. Was this because the two different operations required to locate the lights and keys when they were separated each took about the same time? In six-choice experiments continuing those of Table 4.1. (Welford, 1975), shifting the positions of lights relative to keys produced reaction times expected for a strategy of successive dichotomising. Are more efficient strategies difficult to attain without substantial compatibility between display and response? Perhaps, as the strongest challenge, we may ask whether it was a mere coincidence that the mean of the reaction times in the top line of Figure 4.3, where pairs of lights had been transposed, was almost exactly two inspection times longer than the mean of those in the line below where relationships between lights and keys were direct?

Practice and familiarity

Reaction times have been found to shorten, and the absolute differences between different degrees of choice to lessen, after long practice. Indeed Mowbray and Rhoades (1959) claimed that with sufficient practice, two- and four-choice reaction times could become identical, although this result is suspect because subjects were permitted twice as much practice with four-choice as with two. Other studies have shown clear reductions with practice in the slope relating degree of choice to reaction time—that is of K in Equations 4.1, 4.2, and 4.6, and of b in Equation 4.5 (e.g., Merkel, 1885; Knight, 1967; Teichner & Krebs, 1974). The effect is not confined to manual responses, but has also been found for repeating nonsense syllables drawn at random from sets of different sizes (Davis et al., 1961a).

All these results show that practice increases the rate of dealing with higher degrees of choice, implying that some of the work done by the translation mechanism has been saved. How this is achieved is not known for certain. Some of the changes in reaction times seem far too great to be accounted for by a change in strategy of search. It seems more likely that the connections between various identifications and their corresponding responses have become somehow "built into" the operations of the translation mechanism, and are thus ready for immediate use instead of having to be recalculated with each trial. It is reasonable to imagine these connections as recorded in the store feeding into the translation mechanism, as tentatively shown in Figure 1.1. The amount of practice required to attain such storage seems to differ according to the relationships concerned. For example, Brebner (1973) noted that practice reduces the effect of incompatible relationships between hand and response sooner than between signal and response. The process can, perhaps, be thought of as much like the formation of a conditioned response. The analogy is even closer in that the effect of practice tends to be, like the conditioned response, highly specific to particular conditions (e.g., Lamb & Kaufman, 1965; Kaufman & Levy, 1966).

If it is true that translations become "built in" with practice, we should expect reaction time to differ little with degree of choice when connections between signal and response are very familiar, such as speaking the names of letters or digits shown visually. A comparison of familiar with less familiar couplings is shown in the results obtained by Brainard et al. (1962; see also Teichner & Krebs, 1974) and set out in Table 4.3. The most familiar coupling between signal and response, shown on the bottom line, produced a much higher rate of transfer of information than any of the others.

Further insight into such effects of familiarity comes from results obtained by Fitts and Switzer (1962). They found that mean times to repeat digits projected on a screen rose progressively with the number of alternatives when familiar subsets such as 1, 2; 1, 2, 3, 4; or 1-8 were used, but that results were less regular with unfamiliar sets such as 2, 7; 4, 7; or 4, 5, 6, 7. Similar results were obtained when the familiar subset A, B, C was compared with the unfamiliar E, B, P. The latter subset produced response

Table 4.3 *Signal-response combinations used and results obtained by Brainard et al. (1962). Figures are in bits per second.*

Signal	Response	Incremental rates of information transmission between 2-, 4-, and 8- choices
Numbers projected on screen	Pressing keys corresponding to the numbers, placed conveniently under the subject's fingers	5.5
Lights arranged in same pattern as keys	Speaking numbers corresponding to lights	4.9
Lights as above	Keys as above	9.0
Numbers as above	Repeating the numbers	90.9

times comparable with those obtained when the whole alphabet was used, and suggests that when dealing with an unfamiliar subset drawn from a larger familiar set, it is difficult to rid the mind of the unwanted members of the larger set.

In line with the results of these experiments are those obtained for maximum rates of reading. Pierce and Karlin (1957) found that average reading times were closely similar for vocabularies of 16 to 256 common words, and this fact led them and other researchers since to assume that maximum reading rate is independent of the information contained in the items. It seems very possible, however, that it is difficult to abstract a restricted vocabulary from the totality of common words. Evidence pointing in this direction comes from two experiments by Conrad (1962). In the first, subjects read, as rapidly as possible, nonsense syllables drawn randomly from lists of 4, 8, 16, or 32. The times taken for the reading increased with the number of alternatives, but the increase was less for syllables with a high association value than for those with a low one. In the second experiment, subjects read lists of nonsense syllables drawn from either 4 or 32 alternatives on three successive days. The times required to read the lists decreased markedly between the first day and the third, and the difference of times for the two lists also decreased although it remained appreciable. In contrast, the times taken to read familiar three-letter words diminished little and the times for lists drawn from 4 and 32 alternatives were closely similar.

Relationships between controls and their effects

The principles of compatibility between display and control also apply to relationships between controls and their effects, and both are obviously facets of the same problem. In the case of display and control, subjects are conceived of as translating from what they perceive on the display to an appropriate responding action; with control and effect, subjects must relate action to its observed or expected effects on a display. The evidence in this area has been reviewed by Mitchell and Vince (1951), Murrell (1957, 1965), and Loveless (1962). The general principles involved fall broadly into three classes:

1. *Arbitrary rules.* Conventions, such as that knobs are turned clockwise to increase the intensity of a sound or light (Bradley, 1959), lead to an obvious economy of decision and freedom from uncertainty and possible confusion. Many such conventions, or "population stereotypes," become deeply ingrained. They are, however, arbitrary and may differ from one country to another, as, for example, the "on" and "off" positions of electric switches, or from one context to another, as with a water faucet, which is turned counterclockwise instead of clockwise to increase flow.
2. *Seemingly "natural" linkages.* Many expectations about the effects of controls appear to assume a simple linkage between perception and action similar to that of the ordinary coordination between hand and eye, and several arrangements of display and control seem to be easier to operate if they are deliberately conceived of by the subject in these terms (Abbey, 1964). An example of such a simple linkage is that moving a lever in a given direction is expected to move the pointer on a linear scale in the same direction, as shown in Figure 4.5 A and B. Other expectations seem to assume a simple mechanism connecting control and display. Thus, where the pointer on a linear scale is controlled by a knob, the tendency is to assume that the pointer moves in the same direction as the part

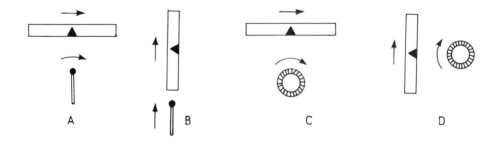

Figure 4.5. *Expected relationships between the movements of controls and displays. Movements of the levers and knobs are expected to produce corresponding movements of the pointers in the directions indicated by the arrows.*

of the knob nearest the scale, as if the two were geared together by a rack and pinion (Figure 4.5 C and D).

"Unnatural" linkages seem to affect subjects of high intelligence less than those of lower (Mitchell & Vince, 1951). Also, their effects tend to be less with continuous tracking tasks where the subject is constantly making movements so that each can be made with reference to the one preceding, than when only occasional adjustments are required. Effects are reduced by training, but are not entirely eliminated, as is shown by the fact that confusion from unexpected relationships may occasionally occur even with well-practiced subjects, especially under conditions of stress (Taylor & Garvey, 1959).

3. *"Mental models."* The linkages between single displays and controls shade into more elaborate conceptual models which enable the various parts of a machine or industrial plant to be related and conceived of as a unified whole. We have already referred to such models at the end of Chapter 3 as similar to the spatial frameworks of everyday perception. It must be emphasized, however, that they seem also to codify a set of related responses. Like the perceptual frameworks already discussed, the models need not be strictly accurate in order to be useful. The model conceived by the operator of an industrial plant is often crude and grossly inaccurate, but it enables the person to coordinate the individual items of the task so that they appear less arbitrary than they otherwise would.

It seems clear that these models represent a recoding of the data provided by the plant and by observation of the effects of controls, which is more economical than a set of rules of thumb in that fewer separate instructions have to be carried in the operator's memory. In some industrial plants, deliberate attempts are made to show the essential relationships between different parts by means of "mimic diagrams" such as circuit diagrams connecting meters and switches on an electrical control panel (for examples see Welford, 1960a, pp. 7, 9, and 25). Such mimic diagrams, by reducing the amount of mental model building that has to be done by the individual operator, can be regarded as reducing the skill required by the job.

Sequential effects

Mowrer (1940), in a now classical experiment, required his subjects to respond as quickly as possible to a signal which recurred without warning at 12-second intervals. He found that when he occasionally gave the signal either earlier or later, reaction time was longer. He argued that reaction time could therefore be used as a measure of "expectancy." Several researchers since have found that if a signal is given after a warning and the interval between warning and signal—the "foreperiod"—is varied randomly from trial to trial, reactions are faster after foreperiods somewhere around the middle of the range used. A warning signal is likely to occupy the central mechanisms for a brief period even though no overt response has to be made to it, so that with very short foreperiods there may be delays due to the single-channel limitation outlined in Figure 1.2. This is, however, not the whole explanation, because longer reaction times are found when the shorter foreperiods of the range are used, even though the shortest are far too long for single-channel delays to have any effect.

The changes of reaction time with foreperiod seem to be associated with changes in cortical-evoked potentials (Karlin & Martz, 1973; Besrest & Requin, 1973). These are such as to suggest that the warning signal to some extent preactivates the response, so that it is more readily triggered when the signal arrives. The preparation can reach such a pitch that a strong irrelevant signal can trigger the response; for example, a subject who is prepared to press a key when a light appears may press it if the experimenter claps his hands. Optimum states of readiness appear to be difficult to maintain (Requin, 1969), so that the subject will tend to prepare for the signal to arrive at the moment judged most probable, and the preparation will be less than maximum if the signal comes either earlier or later. The time which is most probable subjectively may, of course, not be so objectively. It seems to be influenced partly by the series of foreperiods as a whole, but more particularly by those in the one or two immediately preceding trials.

This type of preparation can also explain why reaction times are generally lower when the foreperiod is the same for a whole series of trials than when it varies from trial to trial. With a fixed foreperiod the subject can, in effect, react to the warning rather than to the signal and thus has more time than if required to wait until the signal arrives. The danger with such preparation is that if, after the warning, the signal fails to arrive, the subject may nevertheless react as if it had. The fact that reaction time tends to lengthen with fixed foreperiods of more than about 2 seconds presumably means that the subject cannot estimate the longer intervals as accurately as the shorter, and so cannot time the preparation with the same precision (Klemmer, 1957).

Most studies of reaction time in relation to foreperiod have been of simple reactions. With choice reactions, preparation can obviously not be as intensive because the subjects do not know, until the signal arrives, which of two or more responses to prepare. They might prime their responses to the signal thought to be more probable, but are likely to make a substantial number of errors by giving this response to other signals. We have seen in the experiments reported earlier that with deliberate preparation for a particular signal this did not happen to any marked extent (Welford, 1971b, 1973), and that the effect of preparation was rather to bias the *order* in which inspections were made. It seems reasonable to suppose that the effects of expectancy are similar, so that expected signals and their corresponding responses are reached in fewer inspections than they would be otherwise.

Repetition and alternation effects

The buildup of activity leading to the making of a particular response as opposed to others would probably take an appreciable time to die away.

If so, it provides what is at first sight an explanation for the results of experiments which have found that, in a rapid series, responses which are the same as those immediately preceding are made more quickly than those which follow different responses (Bertelson, 1961, 1963; Bertelson & Renkin, 1966; Leonard et al., 1966; Hale, 1967). The effect tends to lessen or cease if the interval between the completion of one response and the appearance of the next signal is increased to half a second or more: presumably any aftereffects of the buildup would largely die away during half a second or so.

Results which link these findings with those of Blyth (1963, 1964), mentioned earlier, have been obtained by Rabbitt (1966), who compared the times taken in a serial reaction task somewhat similar to Blyth's. He confirmed that a reaction was, on the average, fastest when it was identical with the one previous, and slowest when it was preceded by a reaction with the other limb—hand or foot—on the same side. That is, the limb relationships which in Blyth's experiments determined errors, slowed down the responses of Rabbitt's subjects.

Similarity of response appears to be more important than similarity of signal. Studies comparing situations in which each response was linked with either one or more than one signal have shown that changing from one signal to another signal which results in the same response usually has less effect than changing from one response to another (Bertelson, 1965; Rabbitt, 1968). Confirmation that it is the actual limb moved rather than the control manipulated that causes the shortening of repeated responses is given by Rabbitt (1965), who used a multi-choice serial reaction task in which each hand was used for several keys placed too far apart for manipulation by individual fingers. He showed that responses were made significantly faster if the preceding response had been made by the same hand than if it had been made by the other.

It would be expected also that the shortening of reaction times with repeated responses would be greater with incompatible relationships between signal and response and with higher degrees of choice, because in both cases more work might be saved if a new response was partly primed by the aftereffect of a previous one. Both these expectations are fulfilled (Hyman, 1953; Bertelson, 1963; Keele, 1969; Schvaneveldt & Chase, 1969; Kirby, 1974).

Shortening of reaction time occurs not only with repeated responses. In a multi-choice reaction time task where some signals are related to their corresponding responses by one rule of translation and other signals by another rule, responses which are different from those preceding but require the application of the same rule have been found to be faster than those which require a change of rule. This has been found to hold true with verbal as well as manual responses (Rabbitt & Vyas, 1973).

Short-term aftereffects cannot, however, be the complete explanation of such repetition effects, for several reasons. First, they sometimes occur when the intervals between signals are far too long for such aftereffects to operate (e.g., Remington, 1969). They have also been shown to depend not only on the immediately preceding signal but on those two, three, and four back in the series; reaction times become progressively less as the series of repetitions becomes longer (Remington, 1969; Schvaneveldt & Chase, 1969). Second, in some cases with two-choice tasks, repeated responses are slower rather than faster, creating an *alternation* effect, and reaction times become progressively faster as the series of alternations becomes longer (Kirby, 1972). Third, several studies have shown that repetition and alternation effects change if the frequencies of different signals are unequal (e.g., Bertelson, 1961; Remington, 1971; Kirby, 1974). Fourth, Kirby (1975), using the same apparatus as that used to obtain the results shown in Figure 4.3, found that repetition effects in an eight-choice task were much greater for the ring and middle fingers than for the others. Fifth, many experiments have shown repetition and alternation effects to change substantially with practice.

The findings mentioned in the preceding paragraph add up to the seemingly compelling argument that repetition and alternation effects are due, at least largely, to strategies of search which are affected by expectations and by various experimental conditions. If so, it should be possible for subjects to produce a repetition or alternation effect at will in a two-choice task by deliberately concentrating attention on either the signal and corresponding response which occurred last, or on the other signal and response. Kirby (1974) found this could be done. What is the basis of the expectations that affect strategy is not always easy to say. It is obvious enough when there is a clearly recognizable objective bias towards repetitions or alternations in the series of signals. Where such bias is absent, more alternations than are warranted may sometimes be expected, because subjects tend to underestimate the likelihood of long runs of repetitions in random series.

The wider implication of these findings appears to be that the running hypotheses and estimations of probability mentioned in connection with the perceptual mechanism in Chapters 2 and 3 extend also to the translation mechanism in its choice of response. The skills involved are thus not concerned only with the prediction of *events*, but also with the preparation and anticipation of *actions* designed to cope with them.

Summary

In choice-reaction tasks, reaction time has been found to rise approximately linearly with the logarithm of the number of equiprobable alternative responses. This relationship appears to extend also to other types of tasks such as sorting cards. The reason appears to be that when selecting a response, a subject makes a series of subdecisions which progressively select, first, a broad group of responses such as those by one hand as opposed to the other, and then smaller groups until a single response is chosen. Several different strategies are possible in making this series of subdecisions, some more efficient than others. The strategy employed is affected by the arrangement of the display and can to some extent be varied at will. The time taken to make subdecisions can be calculated, and reaction times can be predicted in certain circumstances with remarkable precision. The process of choice is assumed to result in a buildup of activity in the neural mechanism belonging to a particular response. This buildup has a tendency to spread to adjacent responses causing them to be the responses most frequently given in error.

The rise of choice reaction time with degree of choice is greater when the relationship between signal and response is complex than when it is straightforward; presumably complexity implies additional work by the translation mechanism. When relationships between signal and response are extremely direct, as when signals are tactile stimuli to responding fingers, there may be hardly any rise of reaction time with increase in the degree of choice. The same occurs with very familiar couplings such as speaking the names of digits or letters seen visually. In these cases there seems to be a built-in, direct connection between signal and response which avoids the normal calculations made in the translation mechanism. Similar principles of directness and familiarity affect the ease of relating actions to their observed effects.

Reaction time depends to some extent on previous signals and responses in a series. This seems to be due mainly to previous signals arousing expectations about which signals will occur and responses be required next, thus affecting the subject's strategy in choosing responses.

Programming of action

5

The fact that it takes time to react has two consequences which are not as fully recognised as they deserve to be. First, in any developing situation, there must be some prediction of the trend of events because, if action is to be appropriate at the time it becomes effective, it must be decided before the events it is designed to meet occur. Second, any action taken must be ballistic in the sense that an appreciable time must elapse before it can be modified by any fresh information or by feedback from the action itself. These points have been acknowledged for a long time (e.g., Woodworth, 1899), but have begun to gain sustained attention only since the 1940s (e.g., Poulton, 1957).

Both points have far-reaching implications. Prediction means that action cannot depend on any simple connection between stimulus and response, but must involve a more or less complex computation. To the extent that this is so, it reinforces the point made in Chapter 1 that the stimulus-response and conditioned reflex approaches to performance are inadequate. The ballistic principle means that the elementary units of action are essentially timed and phased sequences of muscular contractions and relaxations which are initiated as wholes. Thus in music, the unit is not the single note but the phrase or arpeggio; in tracking, it is the initiation and arrest of a movement; in tennis, a whole stroke, involving both the drawing back and the driving forward of the racket. In all these cases there is again a complex computation based not only upon the immediate stimulus to action, but upon future goals, past experiences, and concurrent factors such as posture at the moment of action. Although, therefore, the repeated musical phrase or tracking adjustment or particular type of tennis stroke is in one sense the same as those executed previously, in another sense it is never the same.

Reaction time makes it necessary that these principles apply over a fraction of a second, but they seem to operate also on much longer time scales.

For example, in order to find a room in an office building we have never visited before, we may have to predict its position from observing room numbers around the point at which we enter, and to climb stairs and traverse corridors over a substantial distance before obtaining information which confirms or denies the rightness of what we have done. On an even longer scale, every research worker knows that the planning, execution, and publishing of a piece of research involves predictions and lines of action which often extend over months or years before modification in the light of results becomes possible. While, therefore, attention has usually been concentrated on very short-term programs of action, one should remember, in order to keep perspective, that much longer-term programs have also to be considered. It seems, in fact, possible to think of units of action in the same way as the units of perception discussed in Chapter 3; they form a hierarchy in time, ranging from simple actions such as moving a finger to press a key, all the way through to lines of work and endeavor which extend over a lifetime and can be regarded as the basis of many facets of personality.

Saying this, however, immediately raises a number of questions, especially; What determines the size of the programmed unit? To what extent is the size of the unit modified by training? What is the nature and basis of timing in sequential action? We shall attempt answers to these questions in turn.

Size of unit

Factors which affect length of program appear to fall into two distinct classes: on the one hand are those which determine the minimum duration of unit necessary if performance is to match events, and on the other are those which set maximum limits to coherence. Most programs probably lie between these limits, and for them the question is, what determines size. To answer this, we need to consider several lines of work concerned with the control of movement.

Time required to modify action

This obviously depends upon the time that must elapse before any new information signalling that modification of action is required can become effective. It will thus vary with anything which affects the reaction time to such modifying signals. It will be lengthened by requirements for fine discrimination, wide degrees of choice or high criteria of accuracy. It will be shortened by expectations which enable some of the discrimination and choice required to be done before the signal arrives, by efficient strategies which minimize the process of search among alternatives, and by risky criteria of decision which condone a high rate of error. It will be affected in these ways not only by the processes required to deal with the signal immediately concerned, but by any processes dealing with previous signals which, owing to the single-channel effects mentioned in Chapter 1, must be completed before those required by the present signal can begin. In short, the time will depend upon the amount of central "work" to be done before the signal can be identified and related to an appropriate response.

Brief movements, therefore, are completed without any possibility of modification. The most striking illustration of this known to the writer arose from a Siamese cat that belonged to a friend. It had the habit of sitting on the shoulder of anyone eating and of pawing at his hand as he raised a forkful of food to his mouth. The result was that the food was deflected into the cat's mouth, and the diner could not prevent this happening unless he moved his arm very slowly and deliberately.

Crossman and Goodeve (1963) obtained the same type of result experimentally by having subjects move a rotating knob to bring a pointer to a target and adding aiding or opposing forces during the course of the movement. The effects were to cause overshoots and undershoots respectively. After a little practice, subjects attempted to minimize these errors by tensing the muscles being used—the effort was presumably to check and control these muscles with opposing simultaneous contractions so that the disturbing forces would have proportionately smaller effects.

Duration and accuracy of movement
Figure 5.1 shows that the accuracy of movements lasting less than about 0.4 second differs little whether or not subjects close their eyes while their hands are in motion. This implies that there is no current visual control of movements over this period (Woodworth, 1899; Vince, 1948b). Movements can, of course, be made at higher speeds than this, but such rapid movements are not adjusted for accuracy individually. For example, Vince (1948b) found that up-and-down movements of the hand made at a rate of about seven per second fell short of their target or went beyond it in groups. It appeared that although the motor system was making a series of phased muscular contractions and relaxations about seven times per second, these were monitored by a much slower control which initiated adjustments at a rate of only about two per second. The program initiated in the central effector mechanism must therefore have lasted at least half a second.

Rapid movements aimed at a particular *extent*, such as rapid to-and-fro motions of the forearm, show a period of acceleration and a similar period of deceleration which normally shade into one another in such a way that if distance traveled is plotted against time, the resulting curve looks roughly like a normal ogive (Crossman & Goodeve, 1963). However, when movements are aimed at a *target*, the final deceleration takes much longer so that most of the movement time is spent on the last part of the travel (Annett et al., 1958). There appear to be minor accelerations and decelerations during these

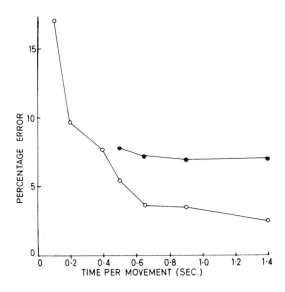

Figure 5.1. *Relations between accuracy and duration of movements with eyes open (○) and with eyes closed as soon as movement began (●). The movements were made by pulling a cord attached to a pointer which moved downwards over the surface of a smoked drum to a target line 1 inch away. The pointer was returned to its starting position by spring tension. Movements were made in time with a metronome.*

aimed movements which suggest that they are made up of a series of impulses each lasting about 100 msec.

The distances covered by these impulses become progressively shorter: the first covers about the first half of the distance from the starting point to the target area, the second covers the next quarter of the distance, the third the next eighth, and so on until the movement can terminate within the target limits. This succession of impulses appears to be programmed as a whole. Crossman and Goodeve (1963) found that it still appeared when the movement was the rotation of a pointer to within an indicated zone on a dial, and the pointer disappeared from view for the whole time between the starting point and the target. It seems that the translation mechanism gave an order to bring the pointer to rest within a given target area, and that the central effector mechanism carried out this order, making minor adjustments about ten times a second until sufficient accuracy had been achieved. It seems clear, however, from Figure 5.1 that visual control is used in movements of about half a second or longer if it is available. We must, therefore, assume that motor programs can be set up which are flexible in the sense of being subject to some modification of detail as they are run through, without being radically changed.

The time taken to make a continuous series of movements between two targets alternately can be expressed approximately as a linear function of the logarithm of the ratio of the distance between the targets to their widths (Fitts, 1954). Those who have studied the relationship have produced several slightly different formulas (for reviews see Keele, 1968; Welford, 1968). The formula that expresses the relationship best appears to be

$$\text{Movement Time} = K \log \left(\frac{A + 1/2\,W}{W} \right)$$

$$= K \log \left(\frac{A}{W} + .5 \right) \tag{5.1}$$

where A is the distance between the centers of the two targets and W is the width of the targets. This formulation regards the subject as being called upon to distinguish between the distances to the nearest and farthest edges of the target to which he is moving, and makes movement time depend upon a kind of Weber fraction. Equation 5.1 gives a more accurate picture if A is taken as the distance between the centers of the actual observed scatters of shots on the two targets, and W as the mean width of the scatters, ignoring any wildly deviant shots. This equation fits reasonably well not only data from tapping alternately on two targets, but also data from tasks such as fitting pins into holes, when W is taken as the difference of diameter between pin and hole.

An example of tapping data is given in Figure 5.2. The fit by Equation 5.1 is quite good, but there are some appreciable, and seemingly systematic, deviations from strict linearity—if the points for the same target at different distances are joined, the slopes are flatter than if the points for different targets at the same distance are joined. This suggests that two control processes or phases should perhaps be distinguished: a faster distance-covering phase and a slower phase of "homing" on to the target. It seems reasonable to regard the former as similar in speed to that of a ballistic movement of a given amplitude and the latter as implying an additional process of visual control. If so, the appropriate equation would be of the type

$$\text{Movement time} = a \log A + b \log \frac{1}{W} \tag{5.2}$$

where a and b are the slope constants for amplitudes and targets respectively. Since ballistic movements show substantial accuracy without current visual control we should probably write in place of Equation 5.2

$$\text{Movement time} = a \log \frac{A}{W_o} + b \log \frac{W_o}{W}$$

$$= a \log A - b \log W + (b - a) \log W_o \tag{5.3}$$

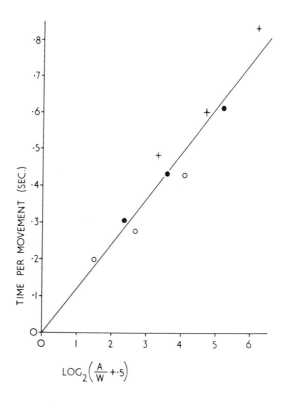

Figure 5.2. *Times for reciprocal tapping between two targets plotted in terms of Equation 5.1.* ○ = 32 mm targets; ● = 11 mm targets; + = 4 mm targets. *The distances from the center of one target to the far edge of the other for each target width are, from left to right, 50, 142, and 402 mm.*

when W_o is the scatter of shots for ballistic movements of amplitude A. There is evidence that the accuracy with which ballistic movements are made is independent of their extent, depending upon some absolute appreciation of end position rather than upon distance moved (Keele & Ells, 1972; Marteniuk & Roy, 1972; Marteniuk et al., 1972; Laabs, 1974; Paillard & Brouchon, 1974). If so, W_o can be taken as constant.

The data from Figure 5.2 plotted in terms of Equation 5.3 are shown in Figure 5.3. It can be seen that the fit is good except for the point farthest to the left. The time taken by short movements between wide targets is commonly longer than predicted in tasks of this kind, and it seems as if there is some minimum duration of aimed movements below which they do not fall, no matter how little demand is made for accuracy. An estimate of W_o can be obtained from Figure 5.3, since the distance from zero to the point where the regression line cuts the abscissa = $(b - a) \log W_o$. In the example shown, W_o worked out at 24 mm, which is certainly of the

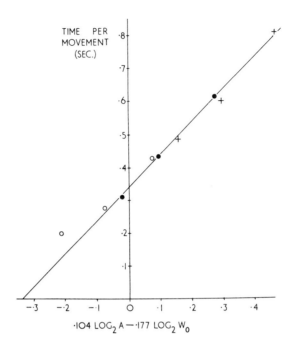

TIME PER MOVEMENT (SEC.)

·104 LOG$_2$ A — ·177 LOG$_2$ W$_0$

Figure 5.3. *The same data as in Figure 5.2 plotted in terms of Equation 5.3. The regression line cuts the abscissa at (b − a) log W$_0$. The value corresponds to a W$_0$ of 24 mm.*

right order of magnitude. The rates of gain of information implied by the slope constants *a* and *b* are respectively 9.6 bits per second and 5.6 bits per second. The latter is close to that found by Hick (1952a) and others for choice reaction times. One may suppose that the first rate of gain represents the capacity of the effector mechanism, and that the second represents control involving the translation mechanism.

It should be noted that the velocity of aimed movements made at maximum speed rises with amplitude. For example, El-Temamy (1966), using a weight which slid back and forth on a rod, found that the time taken for any given degree of accuracy rose by only about 30 percent as the weight was increased from 1.25 to 12 pounds. It can be argued that the rise is likely to be small because the arm itself is a large element in the total mass to be moved, but close examinations by Taylor and Birmingham (1948) of tracking performance and by El-Temamy of his results made it clear that the force deployed rose considerably with heavier weights and larger amplitudes. Had the same forces been used with lighter weights or shorter amplitudes, the movements would have been considerably faster. It seems, in fact, that with increased amplitude or load the subject increases the force applied while keeping the time roughly constant. This, of course, is what would be expected if the limiting factor was the time required to process the data on which control was based. Additional support for this general view comes from the well-recognized fact that complex movements involving a series of different directions or extents, thus implying more elaborate control, take substantially longer to execute than do simple linear movements (Woodworth, 1899; Peters & Wenborn, 1936) and also from the finding that speed of arm movement has little to do with the strength or effective mass of the arm (Pierson, 1961).

Correction of errors

The times taken to correct errors seem to vary widely. Some are as long as normal reaction times in the task concerned; others are much shorter (e.g., Gibbs, 1965). The model outlined in Figure 1.1 and the discussions in preceding chapters make it understandable why this is so. We have conceived of the central effector stage of Figure 1.1 as being triggered by orders from the translation mechanism based on information supplied by the perceptual mechanism. Errors might occur at any of the three stages, and the time taken to correct them would vary with the stage at which they occurred. Consider, for example, errors in making a tracking movement. One possibility is that observation of the misalignment between target and pointer has been faulty, in which case all three stages will be involved in rectifying the error, and the time taken will be of the same order as that for a normal reaction. Alternatively, it may be that the misalignment was correctly perceived, but an inappropriate action was chosen. In this case, further work will be required in the second and third stages only, and the time taken to rectify the error will be correspondingly shorter. It may be shorter still if the error is confined to the third stage; in this situation no new "orders" are required either from the first stage to the second or from the second to the third, and the only modification needed will be within the third stage. Classification of errors in a similar way has been discussed by Rabbitt (1967), and by Rabbitt and Vyas (1970).

How errors are detected is another matter. Presumably some feedback from the response does not match the orders given by the first or second stages (e.g., Adams, 1971; Schmidt & White, 1972). Models have usually included separate feedback loops from responding members to all previous stages, but it is questionable whether this assumption is necessary. Feedback to the first stage should be sufficient if it can be assumed that when the first or second stages do not have new work to do, they take virtually no time to operate. The question seems to be open to experimental attack since, although these stages might operate instantaneously if clear, they would be unlikely to do so if occupied in dealing with other signals. In this case, we might expect that correction of errors, even of those originating in the third stage, would be subject to delays resulting from single-channel operation as indicated in Figure 1.2. Such delays should not occur if every stage has its own feedback loop.

Speed of continuous performance

Delays in responding due to single-channel limitations seem to occur not only when a signal for action arises during the reaction time to a previous signal, as indicated in Figure 1.2, but also when signals arrive during or shortly after the response to a previous signal. The reason appears to be that subjects tend spontaneously to monitor their responses. In our present terms, feedback from significant points in the response, especially the beginning and the end, tends to monopolize the perceptual and translation mechanisms for brief periods during which other signals cannot be dealt with. For simple hand movements, such as pressing a key or moving a lever to track a target, the time for which either the beginning or the end of a movement captures the single channel is about .15 to .2 second. It may well be asked why delays due to monitoring do not also occur when a signal arrives during the reaction time to a previous signal. The reason is, presumably, that signals from the outside have priority and tend to suppress attention to monitoring if they are waiting to be dealt with when the gate to the translation mechanism is opened. We shall note some experimental evidence in favor of this view later.

Meanwhile, it follows that in a continuous task, such as tracking a moving target, the maximum speed at which adjustments can be made will depend on the sum of the times taken by the slowest of the central mechanisms—usually the translation mechanism—to deal with signals from outside and to monitor responses. How much time is taken by the latter will depend on the following circumstances:

(a) When actions have to be carried out meticulously and the display is static, as for example when tracing carefully over a pattern, subjects may well monitor the ends of movements as well as any earlier significant points.

(b) When action does not have to be so precise, or when the display is changing so that misalignments are continually building up, only the beginnings of movements are likely to be monitored. With a reaction time of about .3 second, and a monitoring time of .2 second, successive adjustments would be made at about half-second intervals, as has been found to occur in tracking tasks (Vince, 1948a). If the track changes direction more frequently than this, performance deteriorates markedly (Welford, 1958).

(c) When the display changes very fast, all monitoring may be eliminated. In tracking tasks this might occur if misalignment built up so fast that there was always a substantial correction waiting to be made before the end of the reaction time to the previous observation. Speed of performance in this case would depend on reaction time alone. Accuracy in these circumstances would, however, tend to be low unless responses were very simple and ungraded, since any error made in one movement could not be corrected in the next, but only in the one following that. This type of performance seems to have been attained in high-speed tracking experiments when the track was changing direction three times per second. Subjects maintained the correct number of changes, but accuracy was very poor compared with that attained with changes of two per second or less (Welford, 1958).

In all these cases, speed of performance is essentially limited by the decision process involved in responding to signals and monitoring action rather than by the execution of movements. Limitation of the speed of performance by decision processes rather than by motor action is also illustrated in several everyday activities, perhaps most notably in speaking (Goldman-Eisler, 1956, 1958, 1961; Henderson et al., 1965). Although occasionally people think faster than they can speak, more often they are unable to formulate the content of a statement fast enough to maintain a rapid flow of significant words. As a result, they may speak slowly and thus adjust the speed of action to that of central control. Alternatively, they may introduce redundant words or meaningless sounds (such as "er"), make pauses, or reduce the average information per word of the statement. Such effects tend to be more pronounced preceding high-information words and in sentences involving difficult constructions or other complex cognitive activity. This is to be expected on the basis that these require relatively long times to retrieve data from memory or to order words in a sequence.

The fact that both data from outside and feedback from a subject's own voice have to be processed, and that doing so takes time, is illustrated in an experiment by Broadbent (1952) in which subjects had to reply to a series of questions resembling military signal messages. Occasionally a question was asked while the subject was answering a previous question. In these cases, errors tended to occur either in the reply being made or in the reply to the message coming in at the time, indicating that the decision mechanism was being overloaded by the task of speaking and listening concurrently. Simultaneous translators seem to acquire the ability to speak and listen concurrently after long practice, but they apparently do not monitor their own voices. Consequently, their speaking voices are often strange, and they themselves report that they have little idea of what they are saying as they translate, or confidence that it is correct.

Interaction of concurrent tasks

The view that has been outlined of continuous performance has implications for tasks in which signals for action arrive at irregular intervals and have to be dealt with as soon as possible. We may take as an example a task used by Conrad (1951, 1954a, b) in which the subject watched a number of dials, each with a rotating pointer. He had to respond by turning a knob or pressing a key under each dial whenever its pointer passed any of several marks on the edge of the dial. The number of coincidences missed rose rapidly as the frequency of their occurrence increased. The omissions did not result from inability to make the number of motor responses required in the time. They can, however, be accounted for by assuming that dealing with each coincidence took a roughly equal time during which no other signal could be dealt with: as the rate of presentation rose, so did the likelihood of a coincidence occurring during the time that data resulting from a previous coincidence were being processed. Coincidences could have been missed when this happened, either because data about them failed to be held in store, or because by the time they could be dealt with the pointer had gone past the mark and it was too late. Treatment of some of Conrad's results in these terms, assuming that signals arrived at random intervals of time, is shown in Figure 5.4. It should be noted that the times which fit the results for two, three, and four dials are in the proportions 1, 1.58, and 2, which are the logarithms to base 2 of 2, 3, and 4 respectively. In other words, the times are in accordance with Hick's law (Welford, 1968).

An important extension of this treatment is to the measurement of the load imposed by tasks which occupy the central mechanisms without leading

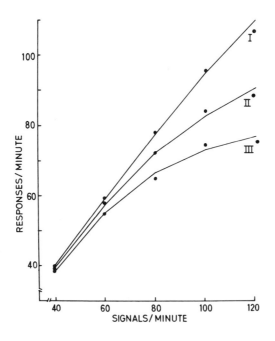

Figure 5.4. *Relationships between numbers of signals presented at irregular intervals and numbers of responses. Conrad's (1951) data fitted, assuming that signals arrive at random intervals and that dealing with each takes an equal time, t. It is also assumed that a signal can wait if the subject cannot deal with it immediately, but that data from not more than two signals at a time can wait in this way: in other words, the latitude in responding is two signals. I: 2 dials, t = .37 sec; II: 3 dials, t = .59 sec; III: 4 dials, t = .74 sec.*

to observable activity. An example is process monitoring in certain industrial plants where a great deal of checking of instruments may be involved, but adjustments to controls are required only occasionally. The time the central mechanisms are occupied in such tasks can be estimated by giving the subject a secondary task which occupies the central mechanisms for known amounts of time, and noting the extent to which performance of this is interfered with when the two tasks are carried out together. Several studies have shown that such interference does take place, and that it becomes more severe as the primary task becomes more exacting. For instance, driving a car has been found to interfere more with mental arithmetic in busy shopping areas than in residential districts where traffic is less dense (Brown & Poulton, 1961; see also Brown, 1962, 1965a, b; Brown et al., 1969).

When two tasks of unequal difficulty are paired, and neither has priority over the other, it is performance of the easier that tends to suffer more (Mowbray, 1953). This is understandable since the more difficult task will tend to occupy the single channel for longer periods than the easy one. Capture of the single channel by the more difficult task would mean the omission of a relatively large block of data from the easier task, whereas capture by the easier task would cause a relatively brief interruption of the more difficult task.

It seems fair to suggest that a parallel to the interference effects in such concurrent tasks can be seen in the effects of worries and preoccupations in everyday life. The absentmindedness, unobservant behavior, and erratic performance which often go with anxiety and unsolved problems seem likely results of thoughts which, even though they result in little or no overt action, occupy the central mechanisms to the exclusion of data from the task being performed at the time. The situation is epitomized by the student who fails to settle down to studying because the central mechanisms are preoccupied with worry about not studying hard enough.

Repetitive sequences

Some indication of the factors determining maximum length of program could probably be obtained from study of the maximum length of repetitive sequence of performance that can be maintained without conscious attention. Controlled experimental studies specifically directed to this question seem to be lacking, although observation suggests they would be instructive. For example, many women report that they can read or carry on a conversation while knitting, provided the pattern is fairly simple, but that beyond a certain level of complexity they have to give all, or virtually all, their attention to the knitting. Analogies could doubtless be found in many repetitive industrial tasks, such as light assembly or packaging, in which operatives are able to talk while performing a sequence of operations.

The length of sequence that can be maintained must depend on the capacity of some mechanism in the brain to take up a succession of different states without their becoming confused or being bypassed. Superficially, such capacity might appear to depend on a form of storage similar to that of short-term memory, and it would seem worthwhile to see whether capacities and other characteristics of the two systems are sufficiently similar to imply a common basis. However, one suspects that the storage of sequences of action is more resistant to the disruptive effects of shifts of attention than is short-term memory for cognitive material, and therefore that the two types of material are carried in different types of storage. Sequences of action are probably carried in some form of long-term memory from which they are recovered when required for use. When in use, they are probably stored temporarily in the translation mechanism as immediate "standing orders" for the performance concerned, separately from cognitive data.

Storage, however, may not be the only source of limitation on length of program. A promising line for research appears to lie in asking why some types of sequence of action are more difficult than others, in that they are performed more slowly or less accurately. For example, when tapping with the fingers of one hand, the sequence

Index, Middle, Middle, Ring, Little

seems less difficult to perform repeatedly at a rapid rate than

Index, Middle, Ring, Middle, Little.

A plausible reason immediately suggests itself: the second sequence takes up the same state at two different points. Alternatively, it may be that some *transitions* are more difficult than others. For example

Index, Middle, Ring, Little

is easier than

Index, Ring, Middle, Little,

perhaps because transitions to nonadjacent fingers involve the inhibition of intermediate positions.

If we try to probe this kind of difficulty further, we may note that sequences of tapping tend to occur in short bursts—each sequence of four or five taps tends to be separated from the next by a brief pause. Possible reasons for these pauses are:

(a) The central effector mechanism has to obtain fresh orders from the translation mechanism. In other words, the limitation is in the size of sequence that can be transmitted by the translation to the central effector mechanism.

(b) Taking up a series of states, especially those involving transitions to nonadjacent positions, is likely to cause neural noise in the motor system: action produces aftereffects which take time to dissipate and so may confuse the perception of signals and choice of responses which follow.

(c) Time may be required periodically to monitor feedback from the actions in the sequence as a check on accuracy.

It may well be that all these factors operate. It seems possible, however, to sort out their relative importance experimentally. To the extent that (a) is true, performance should improve as the coding of the units in the translation mechanism becomes more thorough: for example, it should be easier—as indeed it is—to type familiar words than strings of random letters (Shaffer & Hardwick, 1968). The aftereffects envisaged in (b) should be less serious if more responding members are used for any given length of sequence—say the fingers of both hands instead of one. The effect of (c) should be reduced by any conditions conducive to the ignoring of feedback, such as the effects of long practice, which will be discussed later.

Longer-term programs

At the beginning of this chapter it was suggested that, in addition to relatively short programs of action, there were programs operating over longer periods and forming a hierarchy in which the higher members control and coordinate the lower. Thus, in the playing of a piece of music, it is possible to identify not only individual arpeggios but also broader aspects of programming which set the style and pace with which the piece is performed (Michon, 1974). Such longer-term programs must obviously be less tightly organized and more flexible than those we have been mainly considering up to now. They presumably depend upon some form of storage in which more or less sustained biases can be held for the selection and interpretation of incoming data, and for the choice and shaping of action. The degree of flexibility attained can plausibly be related to the capacity of such storage. If the capacity is small, only the central aim can be held; if it is larger, there is room for a broader spectrum of considerations that may result not only in more efficient strategies of action but in strategies less tied to what is seen as the most direct approach towards the desired goal. It is tempting to regard this problem as being related to that of intellectual capacity to hold a large quantity of data in mind at any one moment, and thus to the ability to see a complex problem as a whole.

Effects of practice

There is a tendency for the spans of motor programs to become longer with practice, probably for several reasons. One seems likely to be that the cognitive units on which the motor performance is based become larger as data in the perceptual and translation mechanisms become better coded. Thus the span of apprehension and the unit of reading aloud increase as words and phrases come to be recognized as wholes. For example, language units increase in length from early childhood onwards, and are longer for familiar material than unfamiliar, and in one's native language than in an imperfectly acquired second language. Such improved coding would tend to shorten the time it takes to process data, and would thus cut down interference effects when signals arrive in rapid succession or when two tasks have to be performed simultaneously. Improved coding would also tend to improve accuracy, so that less time would be spent correcting errors. The effects would be especially marked if translations from perception to action for highly familiar material came to be "built-in," as suggested in Chapter 4.

To what extent there are analogous effects of practice on the motor side is not entirely clear, but it is well known that thoroughly practiced actions tend to become "automatic" in the sense that they are performed without conscious control. It is often held that this implies a bypassing of the translation mechanism, and possibly of the perceptual mechanism also, but this seems questionable. Genuine bypassing of these mechanisms would imply that other signals could be processed for the entire time of an automatic performance, and thus that two quite independent actions could be carried out so long as their motor components did not conflict. It is doubtful if this is ever attained, although it may appear to occur for two reasons. First, two separate actions are possible if they are coordinated in time. The child's trick of patting the head with one hand while making circular motions with the other is an example; the actions are different, but nobody seems able to perform them simultaneously without making the one a unitary multiple of the other. Second, the fact that the earlier stages of the central mechanisms can deal with one set of data while the central effector mechanism is executing a response to a previous set means that two tasks can be interdigitated, with the central mechanisms switching to and fro from one to the other. Two performances executed in this manner may appear to be simultaneous, and indeed are so if viewed on a sufficiently long time scale. Fundamentally, however, they are separate.

It is sometimes suggested that the central mechanisms can genuinely deal with two sets of data at the same time, dividing their total capacity between them and perhaps operating more slowly in consequence, but the evidence seems unconvincing and the conception improbable in view of the seeming unity of action shown by the intact brain. The situation might be different with a split-brain subject in which the two hemispheres are separated: each might perhaps be able to process data and initiate action independently of the other. One can recognize in all this discussion the present-day equivalent of an old controversy which went under the title "division of attention": can attention be divided between two or more unrelated objects, or can it only switch rapidly from one to the other?

A more likely explanation of seeming automaticity than the bypassing of central processing stages is indicated by the results of an experiment by Leonard (1953), in which he compared two serial-reaction tasks. In one, each signal was brought on by completion of the response to the previous signal. In the other, each signal was indicated before the response to the previous one had begun. Performance in the second condition was much faster than in the first, and was accompanied by an uncanny feeling of being a spectator of one's own actions, the actions themselves seeming not to be under conscious control. The likely explanation is that when actions are so simple that monitoring is not necessary, and there is always a fresh signal by the time the response to the previous signal begins, the subject does not monitor his actions, and thus is unaware of them. Such a view is plausible in that the signals were visual and the monitoring was essentially of kinesthetic data: Klein and Posner (1974) have shown that visual data tend to take precedence over kinesthetic in gaining attention.

If this view is correct, we should expect that a similar loss of conscious awareness, leading to a feeling of automaticity, would tend to occur whenever it was possible to dispense with monitoring. This would be especially likely when the coding of the various central mechanisms and the predictability of the external situation were such that actions were always, or virtually always, accurate to within the requirements of the task. They would not require checking for possible need of modification. It is just this kind of accuracy that seems likely to be attained and maintained by practice, especially the continued, intensive practice that is an inevitable feature of repetitive industrial work. The consequences of such accuracy and the lack of monitoring it makes possible are not only faster performance, greater efficiency and feelings of automaticity, but also smoothness in the sense that each action can be initiated without waiting to observe the outcome of the one previous. They will also lead to the appearance and feeling of being unhurried, since the whole time of the central mechanisms can be devoted to dealing with data from outside, and none needs to be diverted to the monitoring of action. Bartlett (1947) emphasized that these were prominent characteristics of highly skilled performance.

One further effect of practice has been noted in the performance of concurrent tasks. It is that the two performances become coordinated, so that alternation between one and the other is orderly and mutual interference is minimized. An example is provided by Kalsbeek (1964) who studied the double task of a self-paced two-choice reaction by the feet to tones of two different pitches, carried out simultaneously with sorting metal rods manually into different sizes. He observed that subjects tended to build up a rhythmic pattern of performance in which the two tasks were regularly interdigitated, and that when this was achieved, the impairment of performance produced by combining them was reduced. Presumably they were no longer separate, but had been combined into one more complex task.

The problem of timing

Of the three main central stages postulated in Chapter 1, the perceptual mechanism clearly integrates data arriving at different points in both space and time into a unified instantaneous pattern. The translation mechanism converts this pattern into an instantaneous set of orders for a series of actions which the central effector mechanism has then to carry out. To do this, the central effector mechanism must transform the orders it receives back into a temporal sequence of detailed, spatial actions—it has, in a sense, to reverse the processes of the perceptual mechanism. The various models and transfer functions postulated to account for human performance have seldom, if ever, really come to grips with the problem of how this timing is achieved, and one suspects that this is an area in which the psychologist cannot hope to progress far without help from the neurophysiologist. However, the psychologist can offer a few seemingly significant facts and suggestions which may give the neurophysiologist a lead:

1. Michon (1967, 1974) has emphasized that the hierarchical structuring of temporal sequences means that they do not consist of mere *successions* of events but of *rhythms*. He notes that these rhythms remain identifiable only within certain time limits—if they are performed too slowly, they tend to break up and become unrecognizable. They presumably depend upon a form of storage with a limited temporal capacity.

2. Martin (1972) has noted that rhythmic structure is found not only in repetitive but also in nonrepetitive sequences. Using illustrations from speech and music, he suggests that the timing and accenting of words or notes in phrases follow definite and universal rules. Such rhythmic structure must presumably apply both to the detailed timing of action and also to the coding of sensory input, since it is obvious not only in performance but also in the recognition of sounds.

3. The timing of any sequence of actions tends to become more precise with repetition. Pew (1974) notes that this may occur without the sequence being specified or coded consciously. He describes an experiment in which subjects had several trials at tracking an irregular course, part of which remained the same from trial to trial while the rest varied. Accuracy increased over the series of trials for the repeated portion more than for the rest, although subjects were afterwards unaware, or imperfectly aware, that any portion of the track had recurred.

4. We have seen in Chapter 3 that the perceptual system can abstract changes and rates of change in space and time which occur in the input and treat them as perceptual data. We may well ask whether there are analogous processes on the motor side. For example, in so-called coincidence tasks (e.g., Gerhard, 1959) the subject brings a pointer moving on, say, a vertical axis to coincide with one moving on, say, a horizontal axis. Is it possible that the perception of velocity is somehow naturally linked, or can be linked, to velocity of responding movement?

5. Speed appears commonly to attach to a performance as a whole rather than to individual components. Thus, for example, if a subject has to set pointers on a series of dials to fine limits—a task which takes longer

than setting them less accurately—movement from one dial to another is slower than it would be if the settings could be less precise. Also, if the subject has to alternate between two dials, one of which requires the pointer to be set to fine limits and the other to coarser, times for both fine and coarse settings are intermediate between the times taken when both dials require either fine or coarse settings (Simon & Simon, 1959; see also Welford, 1958). Again, Smith (1976), in the choice reaction tasks mentioned in Chapter 4, found that when relationships between signals and responses were highly compatible for one hand and less so for the other, reaction times by both hands were intermediate between those obtained when the compatibility for both hands was either high or low.

6. Turning to tasks on relatively long time scales, action which has to be initiated at a particular time tends to be "on the mind" until it is done. This must imply not only that orders for the execution of this activity are stored in some form of memory from which they may be recovered later, but also that some kind of continuing activity bridges the waiting time, alerting the subject when the time has come to act. If so, it is understandable that those who have a backlog of incomplete tasks often feel they are carrying an onerous, stressful load. It would be instructive to consider the nature of these waiting activities and the degree to which their time scale can vary. A possible area in which they might initially be studied is the strategic deployment of effort by athletes in a long race (Ward, 1950). What factors determine the conservation of energy in the early stages and the timing of the final spurt?

Motor processes have been somewhat of a Cinderella in psychology until the last few years. Partly, no doubt, this has been because they are difficult to introspect when they become skilled—that is, at the very point where they become most interesting. Mainly, however, it seems as if the necessary conditions for their study have been lacking. Scientific advances commonly come from a conjunction of interest in a problem and a technique for solving it. Interest in the high-speed motor skills practiced in industry has been strong since before the turn of the century, but the methods of recording fast movements in a continuous sequence were unsatisfactory, and the records were excessively laborious to analyze. The problems of recording and analysis were substantially solved in the early 1950s with the advent of machines which enabled events and times between events to be punched in rapid sequence on paper tape, which could then be fed into an electronic computer (N. T. Welford, 1952). However, by this time industrial interest had switched from high-speed manual work to the potential human problems involved in automation.

The present wave of interest in motor performance seems to have come largely from the interest in sport and athletics noted at the beginning of Chapter 1, and this has brought some lively thinking by fresh minds on long-neglected problems. We may perhaps hope that if an understanding can be gained of motor programs lasting a matter of seconds, we may gain valuable leads to an understanding of the mechanisms behind the potentially more important and interesting programs of action which operate over longer periods of time.

Summary

The appreciable time required to react means that action must be programmed to anticipate future events if performance is to keep in step with a developing situation. The minimum length of time over which such programs operate depends on the time required to modify action after a signal to do so has been received, and thus varies with reaction time and single-channel effects. The maximum length of program appears to depend on several factors, including some kind of short-term storage analogous to, but probably different from, that of immediate memory for cognitive material, and also including much longer-term processes underlying programs extending over periods from a minute or so up to many years. Speed and accuracy of movement appear to depend essentially on the times required by the central mechanisms, especially the translation mechanism, to control movement, rather than on the capacity of the effectors to execute it. In continuous tasks, speed appears to be limited by the times taken by the central mechanisms to process data from signals in the task and to monitor feedback from the actions taken. It is possible, on this assumption, to estimate the load imposed on the central mechanisms by tasks which involve decision but little or no overt action. This is done by combining them with other, more readily measured tasks, and noting the extent to which the first task interferes with performance of the second.

Practice and experience seem to increase the length of motor program commonly used. This seems to be due partly to improved coding of material by the perceptual and translation mechanisms, and partly to increased accuracy of control which makes it possible to dispense with monitoring of action. It is probably this lack of monitoring which accounts for highly practiced actions seeming to become "automatic."

One of the most striking gaps in our present knowledge of sequential performance is the mechanism of *timing*, whereby various actions are brought into play in correct sequence and at appropriate moments. Present knowledge is fragmentary. Future progress seems to need the cooperation of neurophysiology.

Memory and the acquisition of skill

6

In Chapter 1, the development of skill was considered to be essentially due to the effects of practice and experience on the use of basic capacities. Acquisition of skill, therefore, results from learning and can be linked with a vast psychological literature on the subject which extends back to the turn of the century and beyond. Much of this literature has been consistent with a stimulus-response, associationist approach which we have seen in previous chapters does not adequately account for skilled behavior. However, some attempts have been made to link the acquisition of skill to more modern approaches (e.g., Bilodeau & Bilodeau, 1969). Here we shall try to look at the problem in the terms we have outlined in previous chapters.

Experience, and therefore learning, are cumulative in the sense that the way any new situation is dealt with is inevitably influenced by previous experience, and each new experience modifies the manner of dealing with subsequent situations. The modification seems to take the form of selecting, qualifying, and reordering the material held in the memory, and appears to affect all the main links in the chain of central processes shown in Figure 1.1. As regards perception and translation, material becomes more thoroughly coded or recoded, as outlined in Chapters 3 and 4. On the effector side, we seem to learn fine control and temporal ordering of action which can be conceived of as the achievement of a more thorough coding in time. We shall consider these matters under three broad topics: first, the *process* of learning and recall; second, the question of *what is learned*; and third, the effects of long-continued practice.

Stages in the process of learning and recall

For learning to take place and for the subject to demonstrate that it has, a number of stages must be completed:

1. The subject must perceive and comprehend the material to be learned, and select any responding action required.
2. The material must be held in some kind of temporary short-term storage until more permanent registration has taken place.
3. A durable trace which is capable of remaining relatively unimpaired by subsequent activities of the organism must be established.
4. This trace must endure until the time of recall, although it may undergo some changes during this period because of inherent instability or because it is partly disrupted by subsequent learning.
5. A further situation which demands the reuse of the material must be recognized, and the appropriate material recovered.

Let us consider these stages in turn.

Comprehension of the task
Many apparent failures to learn are due to a failure to comprehend what has to be learned rather than to any difficulty of registering or holding the material in memory (King, 1948; Seymour, 1954a). The practical importance of this has been strikingly illustrated in studies of the invisible mending of wool fabric, traditionally regarded as a very difficult operation taking many months to learn (Belbin et al., 1957). It was found that the main difficulty was not in the dexterity required to manipulate the needle, nor in the visual acuity needed to see the fibers, but in understanding the way the weaving was constructed and thus the correct sequence of "unders" and "overs." Trainees were therefore given weaving patterns to construct from elastic thread on frames, and when they had mastered this task they were given specially made cloth with a large weave to mend. This method of training drastically reduced the time required to learn invisible mending of cloth of standard size weave as compared with the more usual method of observing a skilled worker.

Comprehension can often be improved if information on particular aspects of a task is given before practice begins. One caution about such *pretraining* must, however, be kept in mind: although verbal or other information may help a trainee to understand a task, the information will inevitably be formulated in terms of some conceptual model or method of codifying the data and corresponding actions. The efficiency of the pretraining will therefore very much depend on whether the model is appropriate and easy to understand.

An additional factor that can influence comprehension is the speed at which material is presented. If presentation proceeds too fast, subjects will be unable to deal with all the incoming material. They will thus be left with gaps in their knowledge which, in the case of rote material, will lead directly to errors of omission, and in the case of meaningful material, will destroy the coherence of understanding. Furthermore, when lectures and demonstrations are used, it is not easy for a trainee to go back and refer again to a point which may assume a new significance in the light of later information. For these reasons, there are often advantages in using self-instruction methods rather than direct personal teaching.

Full comprehension can be ensured only if there is precise information about what has to be learned, and this in turn presupposes a careful and thorough analysis of the task to decide what should be perceived, what actions have to be taken, and in which ways the latter are conditional upon the former. Frequently, such analysis is difficult because a skilled performer seldom knows precisely how his or her results are achieved, and actions may be so rapid that they are difficult to observe. We may presume that with practice, actions have become accurate enough to be made ballistically without the monitoring of sensory feedback, and that as a result, the performer is no longer aware of them. In other words, performance has come to resemble that of Leonard's (1953) subjects mentioned in Chapter 5.

Often subtle variations of movement seem to appear as qualitative differences to the subject who uses terms such as "keep the ball down" or "follow-through." These terms seem to be reflections of orders by the translation mechanism rather than a description of specific actions, and it seems clear that comprehension of a task needs to be at the level of these orders rather than in terms of detailed movements.

The short-term link

The temporary storage which gives time for more permanent registration has commonly been linked with a form of ephemeral memory which appears to involve a cooperation between the short- and long-term stores in Figure 1.1 (for a review, see Welford, 1968). The capacity of this short-term or "immediate" memory, as it is often termed, is severely limited. Few people can repeat accurately more than about seven random digits or six random letters immediately after hearing them. Of these items, probably three or four can be held in the short-term store shown in Figure 1.1. The rest manage to get through to the long-term store where, however, their retention is still fragile (Waugh & Norman, 1965; Welford, 1968).

If more items are presented, some will be forgotten or recalled inaccurately, although the number retained rises slightly with the number presented (Binet & Henri, 1894; Seibel et al., 1965). Probably a longer list gives more chance for some items to be passed to the long-term store. Such a view is consistent with the fact that the amount retained rises linearly with the *time* over which presentation is spread (Murdock, 1960, 1965). The additional items retained in these cases come from the earlier portions of the list which have presumably been passed to the long-term store. The retention of later items, which are likely still to be held in the short-term store, is not increased (Waugh, 1960).

We shall consider later the influence of skill in passing material from short-term to long-term store.

The amount of data that can be retained in immediate memory depends very much upon the way it is coded; approximately the same number of items can be retained, whether they are random letters or random words each containing several letters (Pollack, 1953b; Miller, 1956). Many more words can be retained if they form meaningful successions, such as a proverb or a well-known quotation. The amount retained can sometimes be extended greatly by deliberate recoding—for example, by splitting up a string of binary digits into threes and calling 001, 1; 010, 2; 011, 3; 100, 4; 101, 5; 110, 6; and 111, 7. Such recoding not only reduces the number of items to be retained but, if they have to be reproduced in the same order in which they have been presented, reduces the amount of information required to preserve order (Crossman, 1961).

Clearly there is skill required in coding and recoding material to be retained, or putting it in a form in which order is in some way indicated, such as by pairing digits, say, 73, and identifying them as "seventy-three" instead of "seven, three." This kind of procedure, rather than any change in basic capacity, appears to account for increases in the span of immediate memory that have been found with practice (Martin & Fernberger, 1929). The increase of immediate memory span with age during childhood and adolescence, and the finding that it tends to be greater among brighter children at each age can perhaps be similarly explained (Jacobs, 1887).

Economy in the retention of order can also be achieved by dividing the material into groups such as "beginning," "middle," and "end" (Wickelgren, 1964, 1967). The effect of doing this is the same as that of dividing items into groups in choice reaction tasks discussed in Chapter 4. For example, a subject who inspected the stored traces of all items individually in a series of, say, nine items would take an average of $(9 + 1)/2 = 5$ inspections. However, if the items were divided into three groups of three, the subject would require an average of two inspections to find the group, and two more to find the item within the group chosen—a total of four. If this approach is correct, the scope for skill in choosing strategies for immediate memory is similar to that for choice reactions.

Errors tend to be greater if material has to be retained for a few seconds before being reproduced than if it is recalled immediately. The reason appears not to be that the short-term memory trace decays with time, but rather that it is disrupted by any shift of attention during the interval, and a lapse of time gives greater opportunity for such shifts to occur. This effect can be very marked; for instance, Brown (1958) found that between five and six letters could be recalled accurately when there was a blank interval of 4 seconds between presentation and recall, but only two or three could be recalled when the interval was filled by reading digits aloud. Disruption tends to be greater when the original and interpolated items are closely similar than when they are very different. Thus, interpolated letters which are phonetically similar to those being retained produce greater disruption than letters which are phonetically dissimilar (Wickelgren, 1966a, b; Dale, 1964). The implication of such disruption for learning appears to be that material will be registered more effectively in the long-term store if the learner gives it time to "sink in" before switching his or her attention to something else; a few seconds or a minute or so seem to be enough.

The phenomena observed in verbal short-term memory have their counterparts on the motor side. These are shown in a number of experiments in which subjects have made a movement, either of a given extent or to a given position, or have exerted a given force, and have been required to reproduce the movement or force after an interval. The reproduction tends to become less accurate as the interval increases, even when no activity is required during it (Adams & Dijkstra, 1966; Pepper & Herman, 1970). If activity is required during the interval, accuracy is further reduced, to an extent which increases with the amount of interpolated activity (Posner, 1967; Pepper & Herman, 1970). Reduced accuracy has been found to result both from irrelevant intervening activity, such as picking up a pencil from the floor (Boswell & Bilodeau, 1964), and from making further movements of the type to be reproduced (Pepper & Herman, 1970; Stelmach & Walsh, 1972). Intervening movements of this latter kind appear to have a biasing effect so that, if they are shorter or longer than the original, the reproduced movements tend to be too short or too long respectively. Their effect tends to be greater when they are made towards the end of the retention interval than when they are made near the beginning (Patrick, 1971).

The similarities between verbal and motor short-term memory make it tempting to regard both as being mediated by the same mechanism. Some support for this view comes from the fact that the retention of movements may be impaired by intellectual tasks, such as counting backwards by threes (Laabs, 1973) or classifying digits into high or low and odd or even (Posner, 1967). However, both Posner and Konick (1966) and Williams et al. (1969) found that accuracy in reproducing movements was not impaired by classifying digits during the retention interval. The latter experimenters also found that the making of movements did not impair retention of digits, and concluded that the mechanisms of verbal and motor short-term retention must be independent. It is perhaps reasonable to assume that they are, but that any severe distraction of attention during the retention interval could have widespread results which might affect both.

Some implications of the short-term link

The very small capacity of short-term memory means that the amount of material that can be handled at any one moment during learning is severely limited. It thus provides an approach to two questions each of which has been the subject of many experimental studies with somewhat conflicting results:

(a) Should a trainee attempt to master a complex task as a whole, or should it be split up so that it can be learned one part at a time? Where the whole task is a closely coordinated activity, such as aiming a rifle or the simulated flying of an aircraft, the evidence suggests that it is better to tackle the task as a whole. Attempts to divide it tend to destroy the proper coordination of action and the subordination of individual actions to the requirements of the whole, and this outweighs any advantage there might be in mastering different portions of the task separately (McGuigan & MacCaslin, 1955; Briggs & Waters, 1958; Crossman, 1959; Knapp, 1963; Naylor & Briggs, 1963).

On the other hand, where the task involves a series of component actions which have to be performed in the correct order, each largely independent of the others, there seem to be advantages in practicing the different components separately. This was studied by Seymour (1954b, 1955, 1956) in the industrial task of capstan-lathe operation. The cycle of operation for this task consists of four component parts. These were first practiced separately, then in pairs, then in threes, and finally all together. The advantages of this "progressive-part" method of learning were small in a laboratory mock-up of the task, but more substantial in the field (Seymour, 1959). The splitting-up of the task in this way enables each portion to be mastered quickly without overloading the short-term link in the learning mechanism.

(b) What is the optimum length of training session? Is it easier to learn a new task by practicing it continuously until mastered, or is it better to divide the time into short periods interspersed with rest or other activity? At first thought, continuous practice seems likely to yield quicker learning because it would ensure that traces were consolidated without the chance of disruption by other activity which might interfere between one practice session and the next. Yet many laboratory studies demonstrate that spacing practice with frequent, brief rest periods is often more effective in learning new tasks. The superiority of continuous practice or spaced practice appears therefore to depend upon a balance between several factors.

Continuous practice seems to facilitate mastery of complex, meaningful material and the establishment of coordinated rhythmic activity. Such comprehension or coordination means that individual items of data or action are grouped together into larger units; in this way, less has to be recalled by rote because more is recovered by inference from one item to another. Also, older trainees seem to prefer continuous practice (Belbin, 1964), a finding consistent with other experimental results which show that short-term memory is more susceptible to interference from other activity among older than among younger adults (e.g., Kirchner, 1958; Inglis, 1965).

Two lines of reasoning have been advanced to account for the cases in which spaced practice is superior. First, if material is indeed held in some kind of dynamic short-term store while more permanent traces are being established, "consolidation" of the trace will outlast the actual presentation of the material and will continue during part of the gap between one practice session and the next. Spaced practice could thus be more efficient than continuous practice if only the actual duration of the sessions is counted and the time between sessions is ignored. This is what most studies of spaced practice have done; when the time between sessions is included, continuous practice is usually more efficient (Tsao, 1948).

The second advantage suggested for spaced practice is that the pauses allow certain aftereffects of previous training trials to die away and thus reduce any adverse influences they might have on subsequent trials. Such aftereffects might well build up with time during continuous practice, and cause interference or noise in the system which would blur incoming signals and accurate patterning of responses. Such a buildup of aftereffects could be regarded as a facet of short-term fatigue which, as will be discussed in the next chapter, can lead to temporary blocking or disruption of performance.

Both factors imply two points about the effectiveness of spacing practice. First, much depends on what is done during the times between practice periods. If these times are spent rehearsing the material, they effectively form a part of the total practice time. Learning will benefit accordingly unless the task is fatiguing, in which case the continued practice may depress subsequent performance (Adams, 1955; Knapp, 1963; Rosenquist, 1965). If, on the other hand, the times between practice periods are spent on another task, learning or later recall of the first task may be impaired, especially if the two tasks are similar but not identical.

The second implication is that very brief pauses between practice sessions should be as effective as longer ones since the kinds of perseverative aftereffects envisaged are likely to last for only a short time—a few seconds at most. Experimental studies have indeed confirmed that rest pauses of about one minute are almost as effective as those of a day (Lorge, 1930). The effectiveness of very brief pauses may in some cases be the reason why continuous practice appears to be as efficient as spaced: when subjects can perform tasks at their own rate of speed, they usually take many short breaks of a few seconds which, though seldom recorded when performance is studied, may be very important in allowing learning to consolidate.

Passing data to long-term store

We noted in Chapter 1 that retention of material learned by rote is improved by active attempts to recite it during learning, as opposed to merely reading it passively (Gates, 1917). Similarly, active rehearsal of material has been shown to improve short-term retention and to make material more resistant to disruption by other activities between presentation and recall (Sanders, 1961). Again, short-term retention has been found to be better if the material is spoken, or even silently mouthed, as it arrives, instead of being simply observed (Murray, 1965, 1966). With motor activity, a movement is more accurately reproduced if it has been made several times before it has to be retained in memory, than if it has been made only once (Adams & Dijkstra, 1966; Posner & Konick, 1966). The reason in both the verbal and the motor cases may be, in part, that active response leads to more precise and thorough coding. In this connection, we may note that Posner (1967) found interference by intervening activity to be greater for movements made when subjects were blindfolded than for those made with their eyes open: the visual data in the latter situation presumably made the coding more thorough. Probably, however, the more important function of rehearsal is to pass the material to be retained through the translation mechanism to the long-term store.

If this is so, data held in memory should show signs of having been worked over by the perceptual and translation mechanisms. We mentioned in Chapter 1 that Bartlett (1932) showed it was not the original data but the subject's interpretation of it and response to it that were stored. Further evidence is given by Zangwill (1937, 1939), who required subjects to reproduce designs or prose paragraphs several times on different occasions and then asked them to recognize the original from among other similar versions. They tended to choose a version based on their own first reproduction rather than the original itself. The same tendency for initial experience to determine subsequent reaction has been found in several subsequent studies. For example, Bilodeau et al. (1964), who required subjects to make movements against a stop and then to repeat them several times with the stop removed, found that the movements made on later trials tended to resemble the first one made after the stop was removed. Again Welford, Brown, and Gabb (1950), who tested civilian aircrews with a series of problems both before and after flight, found that the style of performance adopted by the subjects when the problems were first encountered carried over to the latter occasion. Thus, subjects tested first when they were tired after a flight adopted somewhat inefficient methods, which they used again when they were tested a second time after several days of not flying. In the same way, subjects who were tested first when they were fresh carried the more efficient methods they adopted over to a second test given when they were tired after a flight.

The predominant effect of initial experience is presumably bound up with the cumulative nature of learning. When subjects meet an entirely new problem, they construct their solutions from past experience of dealing with different problems. Once they have done this, however, they have an outline method ready for application to any similar problem on a subsequent occasion. Even if this method is not the best one possible, using it will often be more efficient than working out a completely new method for each new problem.

As we said in Chapter 1, it seems to be decisions rather than actions that bring about learning. The point is well shown in the results of an experiment by von Wright (1957b). His findings also illustrate one of the less fortunate consequences of the predominant influence of initial experience, namely, that any errors made in the first few trials with new material tend to become ingrained. Indeed, Kay (1951), who found this in his own experiments, argued that one of the major problems of learning lies in getting rid of, or in other words *unlearning*, these initial errors.

Von Wright's subjects learned the stylus maze shown in Figure 6.1. The first time through the maze they tended to adopt some kind of systematic procedure, such as always going to one side or alternately to the right and left sides. The second time through, they obviously tried to apply what they had learned in the first trial, making some correct responses and some errors. The pattern of errors made on the second trial tended to persist, so that the positions of errors on subsequent trials correlated with those on the second trial. Teachers of athletics, games, and skills such as typing will confirm these findings; errors should be corrected immediately or they tend to become ingrained.

Von Wright, following a number of earlier workers, argued that if errors could be prevented in the first few trials, mastery of the task should be much quicker. He prepared three different versions of the same maze, as

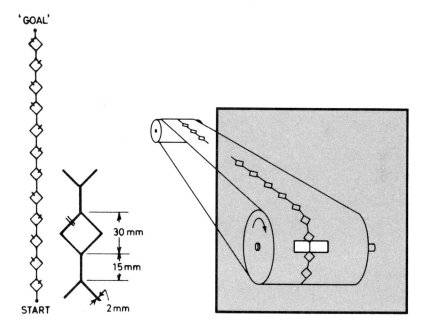

Figure 6.1. *Von Wright's "moving maze." The pattern shown on the left was drawn on a white paper band and appeared, moving downwards, in the slit of the screen shown on the right. The subject had to hold a stylus in the slit and trace over the path of the maze, learning to move left or right as each diamond came into view so as not to cross the double lines on the upper half of the diamond. The double lines were sometimes on one side, sometimes on the other, as shown at the extreme left of the figure. As the subject could not see them at the moment he had to decide which way to move, his only way of being sure not to make errors was to remember the positions of the double lines from previous trials. After von Wright (1957a).*

Stages in the process of learning and recall **107**

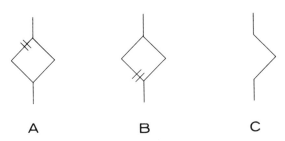

A   B   C

Figure 6.2. *Three versions of von Wright's "moving maze" used in the first four training trials. From the fifth trial on, all subjects used version A. The mean results per subject with the three versions were:*

	A	B	C
Total trials to learn to criterion	23.25	10.45	18.80
Errors made after 4th trial	76.30	15.80	52.15

shown in Figure 6.2. Of these, A was the same as the original maze. B was the same as A except that the bars were moved down to a position which enabled the subject to see them just before he reached the choice point and thus to make the correct choice every time. C omitted the incorrect paths altogether, so that the subject had merely to follow the correct path. Three groups of subjects were used. Group A simply made trials with maze A until they went through twice in a row without error. Groups B and C had their first four trials with mazes B and C respectively and then transferred to maze A on which they made further trials until they too went through twice in a row without error. The results are shown with Figure 6.2: groups B and C learned much more quickly and made fewer errors than group A. The superiority of group B to group C presumably reflects the fact that the former had to observe the bars and make an active decision at each choice point, whereas the latter could follow passively through.

Holding and Macrae (1964), who give a valuable list of references to early work in this field, obtained comparable results using the very simple task of sliding an aluminum sleeve a distance of 4 inches along a steel rod by means of a knob. Each subject was given an initial test to determine the accuracy with which the required movement was made without training, and was then given one of several different kinds of training before a final test. Performance improved less between initial and final tests if the subject held the knob while it was passively moved over the required distance than if such guidance was alternated with unguided attempts or if, instead, the subject made free movements until a stop set at the correct distance was reached. Subsequent work by the same authors has shown that some guidance during training is especially beneficial when tracking movements have to be made where the relationship between display and control is not fully compatible. Presumably, it prevents the errors that would otherwise result from the incompatibility (Macrae & Holding, 1965; Holding & Macrae, 1966). They have also shown that although guidance in which the hand is passively moved is no better than normal practice when learning to track a simple repetitive course, it is superior for learning a more complex course (Macrae & Holding, 1966). This is presumably because errors are more likely in tracking a complex course than in tracking a simple one.

The principle of arranging learning sessions in such a way that trainees must make active choices which are, however, normally correct and so do not lead to ingrained errors has been the foundation of the "discovery method" of training in industry. Its use in training mail sorters in Great Britain is described by Belbin and Downs (1966) and by Chown et al. (1967). Subjects learned to associate twenty village names with their appropriate counties by a programmed instruction method. The program consisted of a series of "frames" exposed one at a time. All subjects learned five villages in one county (Buckinghamshire) first. Then half the subjects were presented with "discovery" frames listing five villages and headed by a statement such as "TWO of the following villages are in SUSSEX, the others you know as they are in BUCKS." Thus, the subjects had to infer the county to which the villages belonged. The other half were presented with further frames listing five villages all in one county to be learned in the normal way. It was found that although trainees aged 20-34 learned about equally well by both methods, the scores of those aged 35-49 were clearly higher with the "discovery" than with the other method and about equal to those of younger trainees.

The discovery method has also been the basis of a series of industrial training studies in various countries including stonemasonry in Austria, the reading of engineering drawings in Sweden, the imparting of electrical knowledge in the retraining of railway steam locomotive drivers in Great Britain, and machine shop work, data processing, and electrical work in the U.S.A. In all cases, except that of electrical work in the U.S.A., the discovery training proved superior to traditional methods, either in the time taken to reach proficiency or in the standards attained (Belbin, 1969).

Retention in long-term store

Material held in long-term store seems to be well preserved over substantial periods of years. It may, however, sometimes be added to, distorted, or overlaid by material arriving subsequently, often without the subject realizing what has happened. This process is well illustrated in an experiment in which subjects were read a short story about a feud between two Flemish families which was settled by a marriage between the daughter of one and the son of the other. The subjects were later shown a copy of Breughel's painting, "The Village Wedding," and later again were asked to recall the story (Davis & Sinha, 1950). Their recalls, when compared with those of other subjects who had not been shown the picture, contained many details which appeared in the painting but not in the story, and omitted many details of the story which did not appear in the picture. Clearly, seeing the picture had a selective and modifying effect upon the material from the story being held in store.

A special but important case of the distortion of memory appears to arise from the act of recall. When material is recalled it appears to be passed through the perceptual and translation mechanisms, and is thus liable to be fed back again into long-term store together with any distortions or modifications it has acquired on the way. A striking illustration is contained in the results of an experiment by Belbin (1950). Subjects, one at a time, were asked to wait in a small room, on the wall of which hung a traffic safety poster. After two minutes each was taken to another room. One half of the subjects were asked to recall as much as they could of the poster. The rest were given an unrelated task for the same length of time as was required for recall. All were then shown another copy of the poster and asked whether it was identical with the first. Of the sixteen subjects who had not recalled, only two failed to recognize the posters as identical, whereas of the sixteen who had recalled, twelve failed to do so.

Retrieval for use

It is obvious that recall involves some process of scanning memory traces to find the one of the item required. The manner of scanning appears to depend upon the precise conditions under which recall takes place. Sternberg (1969a, 1975) has shown that when subjects are given a list of digits to retain, and are then given one digit and asked whether or not it was in the original list, the average time they take to answer increases linearly with the length of the list, implying that it is scanned serially. If the subject stopped scanning when the item wanted was found, the process would be similar to the linear search type of model for the identification of signals and responses in choice reaction times, and the average time taken would be proportional to $(n + 1)/2$ where n is the number of items in the list. With this arrangement, it would take longer to decide that an item was *not* in the list, because the subject would have to scan all the items before deciding, and the average time would therefore be proportional to n. Sternberg found that the times taken to decide whether an item was present or absent were closely similar, implying that, in both cases, the subject scans all the items in the list. The rate of scanning worked out at about 25-30 digits per second which is equivalent to about 80-100 bits per second, a rate similar to those found for choice reaction times with highly compatible and well-practiced relationships between display and control (see Tables 4.2 and 4.3). In Chapter 4 it was argued that this rate represents the speed at which signals in a display are identified perceptually, since the work required of the translation mechanism is minimal. If so, it appears that the rates of search of external displays and of memory are similar. This is understandable in terms of Figure 1.1, since both would be carried out by the perceptual mechanism.

The idea that all the items in the list are scanned is perhaps surprising at first, and has been challenged on the basis that the reaction times for all test items should be equal since the whole list would always be scanned.

Instead, it has been found that reactions are faster to items that have been presented frequently in previous lists (Theios et al., 1973), or that have occurred more than once in a list (Baddeley & Ecob, 1973). There is also abundant evidence that items in certain positions, especially near the end of a list, are reacted to faster than others. The objection may not, however, be valid. It must be remembered that in all the experiments concerned, subjects had to indicate whether or not the test item was in the list by pressing one of two keys, to signify either presence or absence. The reaction time therefore contained not only the time taken to identify the item, but also the time required to choose a response. The differences between items may well have arisen in the process of choice rather than of identification.

Thus, in relation to the results by Theios et al., La Berge and Tweedy (1964) found that more frequent signals were reacted to faster than less frequent, even when both required the same response. Again, anything such as repetition or a particular serial position which made an item more discriminable would cause it to provide a stronger signal to the translation mechanism, and thus produce a shorter reaction time, as indicated in Chapter 2. The possibility therefore remains that, despite the differences of reaction time to different items, the actual scanning process was exhaustive in the way Sternberg has postulated. We could perhaps reasonably expect it to be so on other grounds. The reaction times in Sternberg's experiments can be expressed as a basic time of around 400 msec plus about 40 msec per item in the list. It has usually been assumed that, as each item is scanned, the subject decides both whether it is or is not the one wanted and, on the basis of this, whether or not to continue scanning further items. Forty msec seems far too short a time for this double decision. The times for the choice reactions given in Chapter 4 would lead us to expect that it would take about 90–100 msec. It would, therefore, be a much more efficient strategy to decide in advance to scan the whole list and make one decision at the end, than to make a decision after every item.

The digits used in these experiments constituted a small, uniform, and familiar set of items. With a more complex or less familiar but nevertheless restricted set of items, such as polygons or letters in different styles of type, the time has been found not to increase linearly with n but rather with log n (Briggs & Swanson, 1970; Briggs, 1974; Tolin & Delegans, 1973; Tolin, 1975). The same appears to be true if items are chosen from sets which contain different classes of items such as animals, girls' names, or musical instruments (Naus, 1974). By analogy with choice-reaction models, we might imagine that the subject searches in two or more stages, first in terms of some general feature which distinguishes broad classes of items, and then in terms of more subtle features within one class.

The experiments by Sternberg and his critics were essentially on short-term memory. Turning to long-term memory, Treisman (1960), seeking to explain the results of the experiments outlined in Chapter 3, suggested that words are stored in a kind of "cerebral dictionary" with many cross-references, so that the occurrence of one word increases the likelihood of retrieval of those that would normally follow it. Treisman's model was the forerunner of several other, broadly similar, models of memory which emphasize the fact that any one item, such as a word, carries an array of associations with other items standing in various relationships to it (e.g., Posner, 1973; Morton, 1969; Norman, 1973). We may generalize this approach with the conception that the entire contents of the long-term store are, as it were, contained in a vast array of pigeonholes. The items appear to be arranged so that the members of each class are close together, with the various classes at distances which reflect their subjective similarity. The items and classes can be further thought of as having a mass of cross-connections. Through these, the activation of any one item would tend to spread to adjacent items, and also to some more distant ones. This kind of model is not, of course, meant to be taken literally, but it does seem to be consistent with a great deal of experimental evidence. Perhaps most important, it emphasizes the close similarity between retrieval from memory and the processes of identification, discussed in Chapter 3, which, indeed, appear to be fundamentally the same operation.

Retrieval from such a system involves the selection of particular items, either individually or in a sequence. If so, three implications follow, each of which is supported by experimental results and is in line with everyday experience:

(a) Identification and retrieval should be faster from a small set of possibilities than from a large one. We have already noted that this has been found to be true (Sternberg, 1969a, 1975; Theios et al., 1973). In line with this, it has been found that words exposed briefly are more accurately perceived the more precisely the category to which they belong is specified before they are shown (Reid et al., 1960). We can, perhaps, see the converse of this in everyday life when we fail to recall a name which we are sure begins with a particular letter, only to find later that it begins with a different letter; our initial error has directed our search away from the correct area. It has also been shown that the length of exposure needed for the recognition of common words is shorter than for words less frequently used (see Spielberger & Denny, 1963). Presumably this means that when the category from which identification is to be made is not specified in advance, subjects tend to examine the most likely categories first.

The same principle can account for the tendency, noted in Chapter 3, for subjects to identify successive objects as being in the same class. For example, subjects who identified one object correctly as an animal would try an animal for the next object before trying other categories (Verville & Cameron, 1946). It seems that some continuing aftereffect of identification biases the system and restricts the range of search for a short time. Perhaps the most extreme form of this process is seen in certain senile and other organic mental states. For example, a senile individual asked, "What is the capital of England?" may correctly reply, "London." If the person is then immediately asked a different question, such as, "What did you have for breakfast?" the reply is likely again to be, "London." If, however, a few minutes elapse between the questions, the answers to the second will also be correct—the aftereffect of the first question and answer have died down, so that the answer "London" is no longer in the forefront (Hurwitz & Allison, 1965).

Some indication of the process of search is given in experiments by Wallace (1956), who studied the relationship between identification of designs and exposure time. She found that the proportion of designs identified correctly rose approximately linearly with the logarithm of the exposure time totaled over several exposures. A sample of her results is given in Figure 6.3. The slope varies with the complexity of the material, but seems to be strikingly linear in all cases. The time relationships are what would be expected with a serial classification model operating "in reverse." When the total set of possible identifications is known in advance, the subject selects first a broad class, then finer subclasses until one

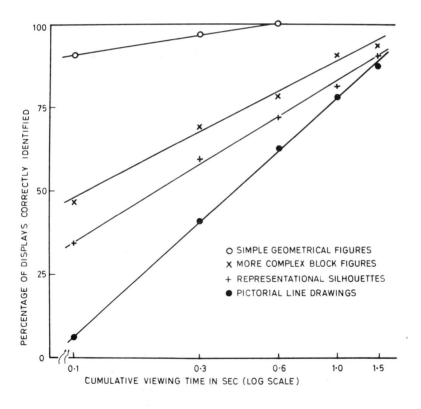

Figure 6.3. *Results from an experiment by Wallace showing the increase in the percentage of displays identified correctly with increase in viewing time.*

sufficiently precise is attained. When the total set is not known, the subject selects a restricted class and runs through it, and then, if unsuccessful, tries progressively broader classes until identification is achieved.

The process of search provides an explanation of the fact that recognition is usually more accurate than recall. The range of search needed to recall, say, words from a list learned by rote, is usually wide: for example, the only limit may come from the knowledge that all the words were of, say, five letters. Recognition tests, however, present the material along with other material, and the subject merely has to decide which has been presented before and which is new, thus, in effect, recalling from a very restricted range. Several experiments have shown that when the set of possibilities is the same for both recall and recognition, both are equally accurate (Davis et al., 1961b; Dale, 1967; Slamecka, 1967).

(b) An important problem of retrieval can perhaps be conceived of as the discriminability of traces from each other. It is obvious that confusion is likely to be greater between very similar than between widely different items. For example, Postman and Goggin (1964) found that learning a list of ten consonant-vowel-consonant nonsense syllables, in which each of four consonants appeared five times, took longer than learning a list in which each of twenty consonants appeared only once.

There is also a considerable amount of evidence from experiments on the rote learning of lists of words or syllables that an important cue to recall can be the degree to which an item has been learned, or in other words, the clarity with which it is registered in the long-term store. For example, the extent to which items from one list learned by rote are intruded in the recall of a subsequent list seems to be greater when the two lists have been learned to the same extent than when either has been learned more thoroughly than the other (Bruce, 1933; Melton & Irwin, 1940).

(c) Many of the facts about the availability of material in recall follow from the concept of cross-connections between items in the "cerebral dictionary." Availability should be a function of the extent to which cross-connections converge on an item and thus on the likelihood of its being to some extent preactivated. In line with this view, nonsense syllables which evoke many associations are more readily recalled than those which evoke fewer (e.g., Postman & Goggin, 1964). Such "association value" is more important than either "meaningfulness" or pronounceability (Lindley, 1963). An illustration of the same principle is that when pairs of words are presented and the subject must recall one member of the pair when given the other, recall is easier if the words of each pair are related in some way (Robinson & Loess, 1967). Less obvious, but clearly emphasizing the role of association rather than familiarity, is the finding by Baddeley (1964) that trivial and meaningless associations between items in a list can improve the rate of rote learning. For example, the pair of nonsense syllables QEM POG was more easily learned than POG QEM, apparently because the letters MP occur more frequently together than GQ in normal English.

Further evidence of the importance of the associative network of cross-connections is the finding by several experimenters (e.g., Eagle, 1967; Delin, 1968a, b, 1969a, b, c, d) that retention is better and recall more reliable when a deliberate attempt is made to form associations between each item and the one following in a list to be memorized. This appears to be one of the techniques employed by performers who entertain audiences with spectacular feats of memory. Another technique, also a matter of forming associations, is to link each item to be remembered to some larger, coherent scheme, such as by imagining oneself dropping the items at different shops along a street. When the time comes for recall, they are "collected" again, from the same shops.

What is learned?

We have spoken about the learning of items and of associations between them, and many facts about learning and memory can be accounted for in these terms. Bartlett (1932), however, showed clearly that an associationist approach cannot completely account for other facts typical of learning and memory in both laboratory studies and everyday life. Broadly speaking, we can say that what we learn is a set of probabilities, that such and such a configuration signifies a particular object, that this event is likely to follow that, and that if one thing is seen another is likely to have occurred at the same time. We can, therefore, argue that the long-term store contains traces of conditional probabilities (Broadbent, 1958). To say this, however, does not really help much. We need to be more specific in detailing what these probabilities are and how they affect performance.

We shall look in turn at some of the principles required to specify the manner in which these probabilities operate and thus cover those aspects of learning which go beyond simple associative principles.

Outlines and details

Bartlett noted that, when faced with learning a passage of prose, subjects do not initially learn it by rote. Instead, they gain a broad outline of the material together with a few details which, because of interest or special significance, stand out. The process appears, as Bartlett (1932) argued, to be the result of perceiving the material in terms of a broad "schema," as discussed in Chapter 3. It is this schema which is recorded in memory although it is typically only an approximation to the data presented. Thus, items in the schema tend to appear in recall even though they were not in the material presented, and items which were presented but are not in the schema are either omitted or may be recalled specially as "dominant details." The overall result of the process is to produce a recall which is both more probable than the original and more in line with the subject's interests and assumptions. Fully detailed rote recall comes only later, if at all (Oldfield & Zangwill, 1938).

These principles of learning and recall of cognitive material also seem to apply to sensory-motor tasks. For example, Slack (1953) showed that mastery of a tracking task began as a general acquaintance with the task and apparatus. This initial stage was followed by adjustment of the velocity of individual movements so that the longer movements were made at higher velocities than the shorter. Later there was recognition of the regularities of the track which enabled its course to be at least partly predicted. It thus seems clear that, in mastering a skilled sensory-motor performance, the subject does not learn a series of movements as such, but a few specific knacks and details of movement set in a broader, more flexible setting of strategies and techniques. Precisely uniform performance, in which there is practically no variation between one repetition of a task and the next, comes at a late stage of practice, and then only under conditions sufficiently stable and uniform that the need for variation from trial to trial is minimal.

Training for skilled tasks is often carried out under relatively uniform conditions. There may, therefore, be a problem of preventing performance from becoming unduly stereotyped, and of preserving the flexibility required for when the skill will be used under more varied conditions. There is some conflict of evidence as to whether flexibility, in the sense of ability to tackle a range of similar although not identical tasks, is favored by training with one example only or with several different examples (Adams, 1954; Callantine & Warren, 1955; Duncan, 1958). The conflict is perhaps due to the fact that although variation between one task and another prevents too close attachment to particular detailed methods, it also tends to impair the subject's grasp of essential principles. Optimum results may require a compromise: for instance, Morrisett and Hovland (1959) found that subjects trained with 64 trials at each of three problems did better when transferred to a new problem than those trained with either 192 trials at one problem or 8 trials at each of twenty-four problems.

Several studies have considered the question of whether information given about a task should concentrate on general principles, or whether it should detail rules of procedure. Generally speaking, the findings suggest that, with very complex tasks, instruction in principles yields better results than laying down a detailed set of rules, while with simpler tasks, a specific drill is at least equally effective (for a summary see Clay, 1964). The reason is probably that a complex task commonly involves a number of alternative sequences of actions, each appropriate to a particular variety of the circumstances under which the task is carried out. Any attempt to reduce this to a drill will mean that several different drills will have to be learned, as well as a system for applying them. In such a case, general principles, even if more difficult to master than any one detailed drill, may effect a substantial overall saving.

Degree of care and effort

Learning a skilled task does not consist only of acquiring knowledge of how to interpret incoming data, what to do about them, and how to carry out manipulative actions. It includes also standards of performance in terms of speed, accuracy, and other factors contributing to and defining overall level of achievement. This point is well illustrated in a number of studies which have addressed themselves to the problem of whether, when two tasks of unequal difficulty have to be learned, it is more efficient to begin with the easier or the harder. Let us consider by way of example an experiment of Szafran and Welford (1950) in which subjects threw small loops of chain at a target on the floor under three conditions. In the easiest, they threw directly; in a condition of intermediate difficulty, they threw over a horizontal bar; and in the most difficult, they threw over a screen the same height as the bar, which hid the target from direct view so that it could be seen only by means of a mirror placed behind it. Different groups of subjects performed the tasks in different orders. The results are set out in Table 6.1: the total error for all three conditions taken together was least when the subjects began with the most difficult condition, and the greatest when they began with the easiest. Moreover, while performance in the easiest condition was much more accurate if it came after one of the other conditions than if it came first, performance in the most difficult condition was slightly worse. It seems clear, therefore, that the best results were obtained when the most difficult task was tackled first.

Table 6.1. *Mean errors made when throwing at a target, in inches per throw. After Szafran and Welford (1950).*

A. Mean error for three conditions together

Direct condition first	5.93
Bar condition first	5.73
Screen condition first	5.35

B. Mean errors for three conditions separately

	PRESENTED FIRST	PRESENTED SECOND	PRESENTED THIRD
Direct	5.59	4.50	4.49
Bar	5.29	4.95	4.96
Screen	6.99	7.16	7.13

Results with some tracking tasks, however, appear to show the opposite to be true (Holding, 1962); practice with a slow-moving, easy course benefits performance with a fast, difficult course more than vice versa. A possible reason for the conflict is that, with a very fast-moving target, accurate tracking is impossible and therefore is not attempted. If this is so, a subject practicing first on a fast-moving target will adopt less stringent standards of accuracy than will one whose first experience is with a slower-moving target. We might therefore reconcile the results by saying that if two or more tasks have to be learned, it is most beneficial to begin with the one which brings about the greatest care and effort towards the attainment of a high standard of performance. Some direct support for this view is given by a finding in Szafran and Welford's experiment not reported in their paper. They found that although subjects who began with the most difficult task were, on the average, the most accurate, they also tended to be slightly slower: beginning with the most difficult task seemed to result in a more precise and deliberate performance.

The relation between aim and result

It was suggested in Chapter 1 and earlier in the present chapter that feedback from the translation to the perceptual mechanism is important in the long-term registration of cognitive material, and that analogous feedback effects, perhaps later in the central chain, may be important in motor learning. Adams (1971; see also Adams & Bray, 1970) has argued that in motor learning of a specific movement, the subject must not only record the "orders" for the movement, but must also associate these "orders" with perceptual data produced by the movement through its effect either on external objects or on kinesthetic sense organs. This is achieved, as proposed in Chapter 1, by some kind of comparison between the "orders" and the feedback data. If this view is correct, learning will depend upon the extent to which the feedback gives clear perceptual cues which the subject can learn. Several studies have confirmed that this is so (e.g., Marshall, 1972; Adams et al., 1972; Adams & Goetz, 1973; Newell, 1974). The essential role of feedback cues seems to be the accurate matching of action to the demands of external situations: mere reproduction of a previously made free movement can be carried out on the basis of remembered "orders" alone (Jones, 1974).

It is perhaps obvious that, other things being equal, the more precise the knowledge given of the results of action, the more accurate actions will become over a series of trials. It seems obvious also that the manner of conveying knowledge of results is important. On general grounds, one would expect effectiveness to be greatest when the information is clearly and simply related to the action concerned. Any distortion or equivocation in the information fed back to the subject will reduce its effectiveness (Morin, 1955; Shelly, 1961; Hunt, 1964). On the other hand, too much or too complex information may be partly ignored (Crafts & Gilbert, 1935) or may confuse the subject (e.g., Katz, 1967). An example has been noted by Singleton (see

"Training Made Easier," 1960), who found that an indicator on the side of an industrial sewing machine which showed how fast it was running, although of some help to a trainee, caused difficulties by drawing attention away from the article being sewn.

What is not so obvious is that the feedback information should indicate the discrepancy between what is required and what has been achieved, rather than merely giving a reminder of what is required or of some broad measure of achievement. The former point is illustrated in an experiment by Lincoln •(1956), who trained subjects to wind a handwheel at a given rate. He found they learned the task more effectively if, between trials, they held the wheel while it was driven at a rate equal to the difference between the required rate and that at which they had been winding, than if they held it while it was driven at the required rate. The point that a broad measure of achievement is insufficient is illustrated by several studies of tracking a target. These studies have shown that merely indicating when the subject has remained "on target" for a given length of time makes relatively little difference to performance (Reynolds & Adams, 1953; Archer et al., 1956; Archer & Namikas, 1958; Williams & Briggs, 1962; Bilodeau & Rosenquist, 1964; Karlin, 1965). The small improvement of performance that does occur may perhaps be attributed to the incentive effect of knowledge of results which we shall discuss in the next chapter.

Feedback, bias, and memorization

The precise way in which feedback operates to affect learning is not certain. If, however, the results of feedback are considered in conjunction with the ideas about perceptual organization discussed in Chapter 3, several suggestions arise which seem able to tie together much of the evidence outlined earlier in the present chapter.

We may reasonably make an initial assumption that differentiated states of the long-term store tend to become permanently established, and do so increasingly the longer they continue without interruption. Such an assumption is in line with the finding that a stream of impulses passing a synapse tends to lower its resistance so that it is more easily passed on subsequent occasions (Eccles, 1953). The more clearly differentiated the state of the long-term store is, the more sharply defined the pattern of lowered synaptic resistances is likely to be.

On these assumptions, it is understandable that, as we have seen earlier, demands for accuracy and active decision facilitate learning, since both would be associated with relatively high degrees of differentiation in the analyzer which would tend to be passed on to the long-term store. With less requirement for accuracy and in the absence of decision, learning might still occur, but more slowly. Data fed back from later stages and from external objects affected by the subject's response would influence learning, not only by the refinement of the biases they would produce for action "next time round," but also as a result of being compared with the initial aim of the action. If the data fed back indicated that action had been successful in reducing the discrepancy between present state and goal, the signals resulting from the comparison would be less intense than if the discrepancy had increased, thereby indicating that some new course of action was needed.

Success would thus tend to leave the states of the analyzer and long-term store relatively undisturbed, facilitating the consolidation of permanent traces, whereas failure would result in disturbance and tend to prevent consolidation. Persistent errors in this scheme can perhaps be seen as those which occur on the way to success, thus forming part of a larger pattern which is successful as a whole, at least to some extent. Thus, if the maze runner who goes down a blind alley eventually emerges and goes down the correct one, the error is in a sense a step on the way to success. Again, the golfer whose poor technique is ingrained may still be a reasonably successful player, although he or she could do better if the faults were eliminated.

The system of biases in the analyzer which leads to traces in the long-term store should presumably be conceived of as some sort of average of the varying biases prevailing on separate occasions. On each new occasion they would form only part of the total system of stimulation and bias which led to decision. Those, however, which formed the common core on many occasions would tend to build up faster than those which varied from one occasion to another. We can thus resolve the difficulty encountered by more rigid learning theories in accounting for flexibility of performance, by assuming that two actions can be regarded as "the same" because they share the same common core, even though the precise circumstances of different occasions mean that they differ in detail.

The present model would account for the learning of sequences by assuming that the aftereffects of one stimulus impinging upon the analyzer would still be present when further stimuli were analyzed, so that the effects of both would be present at the same time and able to influence each other. If so, the model can easily be extended to cover the basic fact of classical conditioning, which has always been difficult to explain. The problem is, how can one stimulus become a substitute for another in producing a response? In our present terms we should argue that, if the effects of two stimuli occurring close together in time tended to produce long-term biases in the analyzer which supplemented each other, the state could well be reached in which one alone could trigger action. In this connection, we may note that in the early stages of conditioning, the order in which the conditioned and uncondi-tioned stimuli occur is not important, and that a response to the conditioned stimulus alone is likely to occur even if the unconditioned stimulus normally comes first (Spooner & Kellogg, 1947). In other words, initially the mere fact that the two stimuli occur close together is sufficient to establish conditioned responding: only later is the sequence "unconditioned followed by conditioned" distinguished from "conditioned followed by unconditioned." This distinction would eventually be made because response to the conditioned stimulus is appropriate only as a preparation for the unconditioned stimulus.

Feedback from a response made after the conditioned stimulus and before the unconditioned stimulus would indicate that the response had been appropriate, and would leave the central "orders" which gave rise to it undisturbed; but feedback from a response made after both stimuli had occurred would signal that an error had been made, and would tend to disrupt the central "orders" which gave rise to the response.

Consistent with this approach is the suggestion by Baker and Young (1960) that knowledge of the results of performance brings about improvement in two stages: in the first, the approximate limits of the action are learned, and in the second, finer adjustments are achieved. What is learned in the first stage survives the removal of knowledge of results, but the fine adjustments of the second stage are quickly lost. It is also understandable, in terms of the present model, that the time interval between the completion of an action and giving knowledge of its results to the subject is less important than the occurrence of intervening actions. Such actions will tend to disrupt the states of the analyzer and long-term store so that they are no longer there to be reinforced by the feedback when it comes. A longer time interval, although it allows the opportunity for disruption by new data entering the system, will not by itself cause disruption, and may indeed help consolidation if the states of the analyzer and long-term store are left undisturbed.

Changes of performance during long practice

It is well known that the initial attainment of reasonable competence at athletic, industrial, artistic, and many other skills is followed by a long period of further improvement during continued exercise of the skill. What is the precise nature of this further improvement is by no means clear, but two points may be noted. First, the data used by the subject may change. For example, West (1967) observed that typists performed better in early practice sessions if they were allowed to see what they were doing, but that vision later gave way to reliance on tactile and kinesthetic cues. The need for such change to take place, if efficient performance is to be attained, may make training procedures less effective when subjects are given indicators to help their performance early in the training which are later removed. The difficulty with such methods is that the trainee may become dependent on the extra cues instead of learning to observe those inherent in the task, so that performance deteriorates when the individual transfers from training to the actual job (Goldstein & Rittenhouse, 1954; Annett & Kay, 1957; Annett, 1959, 1970; Thorsheim et al., 1974; Pew, 1974).

The second point is that, with long practice, changes occur in the speed and detailed timing of performance. For example, several studies agree that if the time taken by a task is divided into movement times and times between movements, it is the latter which decrease more with practice. If, say, a subject has to move his hand to grasp an object and then convey the object to a box and drop it, the times taken for grasping and dropping improve more than do those for the movements between the two (Wehrkamp & Smith, 1952; Rubin et al., 1952; von Trebra & Smith, 1952; Seymour, 1959). Presumably the central decision processes are modified with practice to a greater extent than is the execution of movements.

De Jong (1957), following suggestions made by previous workers, has proposed that the time taken to perform a repetitive task falls exponentially until it approaches some "incompressible" minimum, so that the logarithm of cycle time when plotted against the logarithm of cycle number decreases approximately linearly until it reaches a minimum level. He proposes that

$$T_n = T_\infty + \frac{T_1 - T_\infty}{n^k} \tag{6.1}$$

where T_n is the nth cycle time, T_∞ is the incompressible minimum time—that is, the time that would be taken if the task was continued for an infinite number of cycles—and T_1 is the time taken by the first cycle. The exponent k expresses the rate at which improvement takes place with practice.

De Jong found this formulation to fit reasonably well for a number of industrial operations. The approach was taken up by Crossman (1959), who proposed a somewhat similar formula and found that it gave a reasonably good fit to the data from several laboratory studies and industrial operations. Examples are shown in Figure 6.4. He suggested that the improvement is due to the operator starting with a range of slightly different methods of doing the task and gradually coming to select the quickest to the exclusion of others. It is reasonable to see this as the result of interaction between feedback and states in the central stages and long-term store or stores. The quickest methods are likely to be the least variable, or in other words, those in which the core of similarity is greatest. They are thus likely to be consolidated most over a long series of trials.

Crossman pointed out a number of consequences of his model:

(a) It implies that successive performances of the same task will tend to become more uniform. Some evidence that this is so for tracking has been provided by Reynolds (1952), for throwing by Vorro (1973), and for driving a car by Lewis (1954), who found that highly skilled drivers performed more consistently than less skilled.

(b) Rate of improvement with practice will depend on the variety of methods from which selection has to be made, and the variability of the time taken by each method.

(c) The more subtasks there are in the overall task, and the more they interact with one another, the more opportunity there will be for improvement, and therefore the longer improvement will continue.

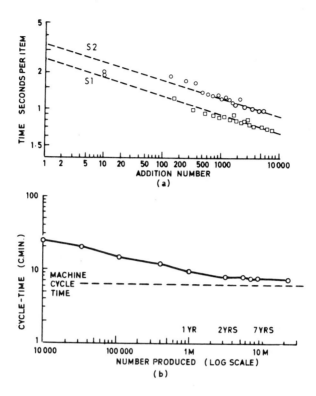

Figure 6.4. (a) Plot by Crossman showing improvements with practice in time taken to add digits. Data for two subjects, S1 and S2. (b) Plot by Crossman showing improvements with practice in time taken to make cigars.

(d) Transfer of skill from one task to another will depend not so much upon the extent to which methods possible for one task are applied to the other, as on the extent to which methods selected for the one are applied to the other. This point provides a rational explanation of the finding by Singleton (1957) that, when learning a new method of work, there was little interference from an established skill among thoroughly experienced subjects, although there was among recent trainees. We can think of the experienced worker as having selected methods so precisely adapted to the old skill that they contained nothing likely to interfere with the new.

With practice, efficiency in dealing with incoming data and initiating action tends to increase. This supplements the reasons given in previous chapters to explain why the skilled person seems to have, as Bartlett (1947) noted, "all the time in the world." The skilled performer has, in a very real sense, less to do than the unskilled to achieve the same end. As a result, the skilled person is less likely to suffer from fatigue, and in many industrial tasks the speed of working will be limited by the machine being used rather than by the capacities of the operator.

At the same time, the means of attaining efficiency may endanger flexibility. Efficiency depends largely upon the attainment of uniformity, whereas flexibility requires that methods should differ according to circumstances. At best, uniformity can lead to a judicious neglect of minor variations between one situation and another, and result in a routine for a job which does not exactly fit the circumstances, but is good enough and much quicker than one precisely tailored to the situation. At worst, it can lead to "rigidity" in the sense that action is carried through in the face of clear evidence that it is inappropriate.

Our knowledge of the effects of long practice is limited because laboratory experiments can seldom be carried on long enough for the full effects of practice to be realized, and detailed studies in industry, where long-practiced performances are available, are very difficult to make. Nevertheless, the questions of how skill develops over periods of years, of what conditions favor the attainment of efficiency and the retention of flexibility, and of how all these matters are related to events early in training are obviously of the greatest importance to all who are concerned with the design and conduct of training programs, whether in industry, in athletics, or in any other branch of skilled performance.

Summary

The process of learning and recall can be thought of as a sequence of five stages:

1. Comprehension of the task. Many difficulties in learning result from a lack of understanding of what needs to be learned. Training techniques aimed at developing thorough understanding have often been strikingly successful.
2. A temporary storage which gives time for more permanent, long-term traces to form. This is commonly equated with an ephemeral, immediate memory which has been extensively studied in recent years. It is of severely limited capacity and is especially liable to disruption by any shift of attention during the period of retention. It appears to carry coded material and has a tendency to retain not only *items* but also the *order* in which they were presented. The limited capacity of this temporary storage makes it desirable to split up tasks that involve substantial amounts of learning so that they may be tackled in portions which will not overload the system.
3. Passing material to long-term store. This appears to be greatly facilitated

by active response to the material, including rehearsal and the making of judgments. Initial responses to new material tend to become fixated, and much of the subsequent process of learning seems to consist of getting rid of initial errors which have become ingrained. Learning takes place much more quickly if these initial errors are prevented.

4. Retention in long-term store. This appears to be highly stable, but material can be affected by other similar material arriving later. In particular, when material is recalled it seems to be "rewritten" in a way which incorporates any distortions brought about by the recall or the circumstances in which it occurred.

5. Retrieval for use. We can envisage material stored in long-term memory as held in something analogous to an array of pigeonholes in which individual items are grouped into classes. The problem of retrieval lies in the processes involved in locating the item required. Retrieval is easier when there are relatively few possibilities, when probabilities can be determined in advance, when traces are readily discriminable, and when associations, either unintentional or deliberate, have been formed.

The second major problem of learning dealt with in the chapter is the question "What is learned?" The answer lies not only in items of data and associations between them, but also includes:

(a) General outline or "schema." This is imposed on incoming material and shapes both perception and recall. Details which are not fitted by the schema are either ignored or are recorded separately.

(b) Degree of care and effort. These have the interesting effect that learning a relatively difficult task may result in better learning of an easy task than vice versa.

(c) The relation between aim and result. Feedback indicating the results of action is essential if performance is to be brought into line with external requirements.

A feedback model is outlined which assumes that data regarding the effects of action are fed back to the perceptual mechanism and long-term store. If these data are consonant with the states there which gave rise to the actions, the states are left undisturbed and thus tend to be consolidated. If they are not, the states tend to be disrupted, so that consolidation is prevented.

Changes of performance during long practice include changes in the sensory cues used and in the speed of performance. Times taken for performance tend to fall exponentially. The fall would be consistent with the gradual selection of more efficient detailed methods of performance.

Stress, motivation, and fatigue

7

Although studies of stress have generated a vast literature in physiology, biochemistry, medicine, psychiatry, psychology, and sociology, it seems fair to claim that the psychologist occupies a central position in the discussion. Stress occurs whenever there is a departure from optimum conditions which the organism is unable, or not easily able, to correct. Assuming this is true, three implications follow. First, since human beings are constituted in such a way that they function best under conditions where the demands made are moderate, performance is less than maximal not only if the demands are too high, but also if they are too low. It is, therefore, necessary to think in terms of both positive and negative departures from optimum as sources of stress, although the former are better recognized, and probably more frequent, than the latter.

Second, as McGrath (1970) has emphasized, stress is the result of an imbalance between demand and the capacity of the organism. According to this view, stress varies not only with environmental and social conditions which affect demand, but also with native endowment, training, and bodily conditions which affect capacity. Sells (1970) adds the further point that for stress to occur, the consequences of failure to meet demand must be regarded as important by the person concerned.

Third, the concept of departure from optimum, and also Sells' reference to personal involvement, link stress to motivation.

The nature of motivation

It has traditionally been assumed that all human motives can be traced back, directly or indirectly, to biological needs for the survival of either the individual or of the species, so that we eat to live, earn to eat, and have sexual intercourse in order to reproduce. Obviously, this view is, at best, only partly correct. We do not do these things for such reasons alone; our aims are more immediate and sensuous. True, it is known that certain biochemical conditions in the bloodstream affect parts of the brain and so lead to hunger and thirst, but these desires may be satisfied by the sensory effects of eating or drinking, long before the actual bodily conditions are restored to balance. The attribution of motives to the biological needs for survival becomes even more tenuous in the case of civilized social behavior and activities such as exploration and play (e.g., Dember & Earl, 1957; Seward, 1963).

Several theorists have proposed somewhat similar ways out of this difficulty. Their ideas are well epitomized in the suggestion made by Woodworth (1958) that the organism possesses an inherent and fundamental tendency to "deal with its environment" and to develop its capacity for doing so. He argued that this was the one fundamental motive, and that biological appetites, such as those for food or sex, use this tendency and are thus essentially secondary. Such an approach has the important implication that motives are linked to abilities, in the sense that successful dealing with the environment depends on the skills at the subject's command (White, 1959). This does indeed seem to hold true, as motives and skills tend to develop together step by step (Hebron, 1966).

The link between motives and skill is, however, more fundamental than this. As we said in Chapter 1, motivation seems to be an essential feature of the operation of the feedback mechanism that underlies skilled performance. Action is initiated by signals which arise when departure from optimum occurs. The signals and resulting action become more powerful, up to the limit of the capacity of the mechanism, as the departure becomes greater, and diminish as it becomes less. They are thus affected by feedback of the results of the organism's activity, being increased if action is inappropriate and decreased as effective action reduces the discrepancy between present state and optimum. Many facts of motivation are directly explained in terms of this model. For example, the actions of a person who is deprived of air tend to become increasingly vigorous as the deprivation becomes more acute, until either air is obtained or physical exhaustion supervenes. Similarly, in many more complex activities, such as problem solving, it has been shown that level of arousal and vigor of action rise with increased incentive, and diminish as a task is accomplished.

The effectiveness of such a system and the rewarding and punishing effects of actions, obviously depend upon the feedback loop from output back to input being closed—in other words, upon the subject having effective knowledge of the results of his or her actions. As noted in Chapter 6, such knowledge and experience not only enable errors to be corrected, exerting in cybernetic terms a negative-feedback effect, but on a longer time scale have an activating, incentive, or positive-feedback effect (Gibbs & Brown, 1956). Stress can be conceived of as developing when motivating conditions are not reduced by the organism's actions, either because they are ineffective or because the feedback loop is not closed so that the individual does not know whether they are effective or not.

Four elaborations of the simple feedback model are necessary if it is to account for any substantial range of facts about motivation and stress:

(a) Action may be triggered not only by the signals which are basically effective, but also by signs or symbols of them. In this way, anticipatory action is possible. Thus, for example, we buy groceries when our shelves begin to look empty instead of waiting until we are actually hungry, and we learn to recognize by sight objects which would be too hot to touch. The corresponding observation regarding stress is that effects often occur before the stressful situation arises, and may actually diminish when it comes. Presumably a person may underestimate his or her ability to cope, and finds the actual task less difficult than feared. Such anticipation appears also to provide an operational definition of *threat* (McGrath, 1970).

(b) Several variables may combine to determine the effective signal strength. In particular, the effect of any departure from optimum seems to be inversely related to the difficulty or unpleasantness of the effort involved in correcting it—in traditional terms, the incentive effect of a reward is partly offset by the cost of obtaining it. Therefore, readiness to undertake action seems to depend upon some kind of ratio or difference between result and cost. Such a relationship provides an obvious explanation of the common reluctance to undertake laborious or difficult tasks. It is probably also the simplest explanation of the fact that, in a task where many things have to be done before a final result is achieved, effort tends to be low at the outset, and rises later as the the goal nears attainment.

The fact that motivation at the time of action depends on the relationship between benefit and cost suggests that stress will develop not only when demand exceeds capacity in the sense that a person cannot cope, but also when it requires effort or the toleration of unpleasantness beyond that which a person is willing to bear. It also implies that stress will not occur suddenly at the point where coping becomes impossible, but is a continuous variable, increasing gradually as demand approaches a person's maximum capacity or willingness.

The same relationship can also account for the varied effects of frustration upon performance. Obstruction to the attainment of a goal will signal the need for increased effort. Provided the extra effort does not drive the difference between potential gain and cost below zero, performance will become more vigorous. A point may come, however, when cost exceeds potential gain and the activity is abandoned. Around the point of balance, any one of several things can happen. There may be vacillation as random variations in the way rewards and costs are seen swing first one way then the other. Alternatively, attempts may be made to reduce effort by changing the strategy of the performance. Again, the goal may be reduced or modified to an extent that, in extreme cases, it is almost unrecognizable, but will at least give the subject *some* result for the effort expended. Sublimation and displacement activities appear to be examples of this last possibility.

One further point needs, however, to be noted regarding the relationship between benefit and cost: although difficulty and the need for effort may make a task appear distasteful, when the task is completed they tend to enhance the satisfaction gained from doing it and thus raise the value of the achievement in retrospect.

(c) In almost any real-life situation, the motives which activate any one piece of behavior are many. To take a simple example, if we were to ask a student in a library what he was doing, he might correctly reply, "Reading this book." He might, however, with equal correctness reply, "This is one of the articles I must read to prepare for a seminar." If we further asked him why he wanted to do this, he might admit that he was trying to secure a good grade for his work, that a good grade was one of the essentials for getting a lucrative job, and that he wanted the job because it was likely to lead on to a position of respect and influence. The reading of the book, the preparation for the seminar, and the obtaining of a good grade, job, and career can be thought of as forming a hierarchy of *aims*, *tasks*, or *programs* of the type discussed in Chapter 5, each on a longer time scale than the preceding. The long-range aims encompass the shorter ones and largely determine the way in which they are carried out. It seems fair to argue that each task in the hierarchy acts as the immediate motive for its component smaller tasks.

Often two possible courses of action, dictated by different aims, will conflict. For instance, a student may wish to prepare for an examination and also to go to a party. In such conflicts it is usually the shorter-term task which brings the more immediate results, and is thus the more attractive. It is not, however, always the more rewarding in the long run, and many social norms, laws, practices in training children, and methods of fostering values and conscience represent attempts to encourage the setting-aside of short-term desires in favor of aims on longer time scales. These regulatory measures obviously do not, and should not, deny bodily needs or the necessity of recreation, but instead, try to control them and put them into perspective.

The hierarchical arrangement of motivation makes it understandable that stress effects can occur on various time scales. Thus a person may cope successfully with immediate moment-to-moment or day-to-day tasks, and yet suffer stress because of feeling unable to attain long-term goals.

Alternatively, individuals may be confident about the longer-term, but be unable to cope with a short-term task. If the immediate task is essential to fulfilling the long-term one, feelings of stress may well be transferred to the longer-term task and have a more pervasive effect on attitudes and behavior than one might expect from study of the short-term task alone.

(d) It is necessary to define what is meant by "optimum," departure from which activates the feedback mechanism. This is a difficult question to answer, but three principles can carry us a long way. First, we tend to avoid extreme levels of *stimulation* and to seek moderate levels. Thus warmth is cheering and cool refreshing, while extremes of heat and cold are unpleasant. Again, a noisy environment tends to be irritating, while complete sensory deprivation is hard to bear. The same principle can be applied to at least some biological needs: for example, we eat and stop eating to avoid the extremes of hunger and satiation.

Second, we prefer stimulation to have a moderate degree of patterning, or perhaps it would be better to say *predictability*, in both space and time. Thus, while most of us usually prefer our clothing, houses, and household articles to have something more than stark simplicity, we dislike excessive complexity. As regards patterning in time, we enjoy a certain amount of change or of the discrepancy between events and expectation we call surprise, but continual unpredictable change is exhausting, and unvarying routine is dull. This last point is emphasized by the fact that conditions of perceptual deprivation in which sound and light are present but entirely unpatterned are even less tolerable than complete lack of stimulation (for a review see Zubek, 1964). Further examples can be seen on a social scale: we dislike, on the one hand, the needling critic who attacks our basic assumptions, and on the other, the bore whose conversation we can largely predict.

Third, we prefer a medium degree of *conflict*, either of cognitive data or of potential action. Thus a person may enjoy puzzles and mystery stories as ways of introducing mildly stimulating problems into a routine world, but dislike making decisions in the face of severe conflicts of evidence or where no possible course of action is ideal.

What constitutes an optimum level of intensity or patterning or conflict may be modified by habituation, as anyone knows who has observed the different volume at which older and younger people play their record players, or the changing styles of hair and clothing, or who has considered the differences between individuals in their propensity to bet or to take risks.

Specification of "optimum" in these ways emphasizes the fact that demand and human capacity are to be conceived of not only in terms of muscular strength or heat regulation or oxygen supply, but also in terms of information processing. In most everyday situations, performance is limited much more by the time taken to resolve uncertainty when making decisions, or by the amount of data that can be handled at any one instant, than by purely physical factors. Some of the most severe demands thus arise from the speed with which a task must be done, the number of sources of data that have to be monitored, or the complexity of the decisions required.

Stress and arousal

It seems reasonable to regard reactions to stress as attempts to secure an optimum level of *arousal* (Hebb, 1955). Sensory stimulation, novelty, and conflict all tend to raise arousal level, while monotonous uniformity, predictability, and concordance tend to lower it. It is also well recognized that performance tends to be most effective at intermediate levels of arousal: the organism is insensitive and inert if the level of arousal is too low, and tense and disorganized if it is too high.

The general relationship of stress to arousal has been described by two models. One, the *inverted-U hypothesis*, simply states that as stress increases and the resulting arousal level rises, so performance improves until some optimum point is reached but thereafter declines (see Figure 7.1). While the model seems accurate as far as it goes, it does not advance our understanding very much. Where, for instance, does the optimum point come? Why does it seem to differ from one task to another? Does performance beyond the

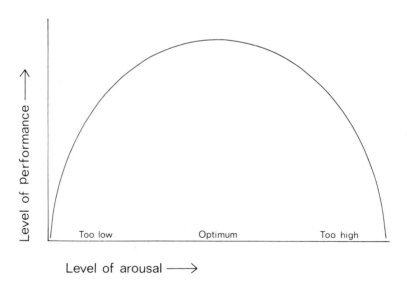

Figure 7.1. *Relationship between arousal and performance according to the inverted-U hypothesis.*

optimum point merely revert to what it was before the optimum was reached, or are the imperfections different above and below the optimum?

The other model is the *signal detection theory* outlined in Chapter 2 (Broadbent, 1971). It has been argued that increased motivation and stress cause the cutoff shown in Figures 2.1 and 2.2 to move to the left, thus raising the number of signals correctly identified, but also the number of false positives.

The weakness of the signal detection theory is that it does not explain why the cutoff should be lowered under stress. This weakness can be eliminated, however, if it is assumed that, as arousal increases, the stream of impulses from the brain stem which mediate arousal partially depolarize the cells of the cortex, thus making them readier to fire. If this is so, both noise and signal should increase with arousal level in such a way as to leave the ratio between the standard deviation of the distributions and the distance between their means—the signal-to-noise ratio—little changed. In effect, both the distributions of Figures 2.1 and 2.2 would be expanded towards the right. If in these circumstances the cutoff point remained unchanged, it would appear to have moved to the left (Welford, 1968). Figure 7.2 shows three pairs of such distributions—one (B) for optimal arousal, one (C) for overarousal, such as might occur with stress caused by overloading, and one (A) for underarousal, such as might be associated with underloading. The cutoff is assumed to remain at the same absolute point in all three cases.

In this form, the theory accounts well for the inverted-U relationship between arousal and performance. Let us assume that the frequencies of

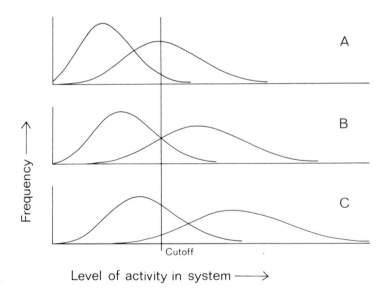

Figure 7.2. *Distributions similar to those of Figure 2.2 for three levels of arousal: low—A; optimal—B; high—C.*

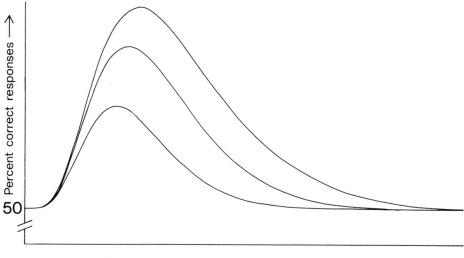

Figure 7.3 *Relationship between arousal and performance in a discrimination task for three levels of difficulty defined as degrees of separation of distributions like those in Figure 7.2. The mean of the two distributions is the same for all three levels. Arousal is assumed to multiply the distributions by a factor which at any given level is the same for all of them.*

"signal" and "no signal" are equal. If underarousal is now so severe that virtually the whole of both distributions are to the left of the cutoff—an exaggerated form of A—all cases of "no signal" will be reported correctly, but no cases of "signal," so that 50 percent of the subjects' answers will be correct. As the distributions move to the right with increasing arousal, more signals will be reported correctly and while there will be some false positives, the former will outweigh the latter so that the total correct responses will rise until the condition shown in B is reached. As the distributions move still further to the right in the manner of C, the proportion of signals correctly identified will continue to rise, but the false positives will rise still faster. If the whole of both distributions are to the right of the cutoff, all signals will be reported correctly and all cases of "no signal" will be incorrectly responded to as false positives, so that the total correct responses will again be 50 percent. The result of moving the distributions in Figure 7.2 from one extreme to the other in this way is shown by the lower curve of Figure 7.3.

Perhaps the most important implication of this approach is the distinction it draws between the impairments of performance by under- and overarousal. Below optimum arousal, subjects are underactive, and their errors are mainly those of omission. When arousal is above optimum, subjects are overactive, and their errors are largely those of commission. Not enough studies of performance in relation to arousal have been reported in sufficient detail to make it certain that these observations are in fact true, but some evidence available seems to indicate that they are (see Freeman, 1933, 1940; Davies & Tune, 1970). Certainly this approach is plausible: the monotony and boredom that result from too little demand tend to produce an inert performance and drowsiness, while the tension and anxiety that accompany too great a demand often lead to actions that are rash and ill-considered.

Similar effects of activation and arousal have been found for learning and memory. Bills (1927) found that if the subject squeezed a hand dynamometer while learning, both the rate of learning and the level of subsequent recall were improved. Other investigators have confirmed Bills' result but added the further finding that if the tension is increased beyond a certain point, performance falls again (Stauffacher, 1937; Courts, 1939). Whether this is due to overarousal, or whether the effort of squeezing a dynamometer very hard distracts the subject's attention, is not clear.

Other findings confirm the general picture of learning being improved, at least up to a point, by increased arousal. For instance, Sherwood (1965) noted that rate of learning tended to rise and fall with arousal level in the same individuals tested on different occasions. Again, measures of skin resistance taken during learning a list of nonsense syllables have shown that resistance differs at different points in the list and that the resistance levels correspond closely to the speed at which particular syllables are learned—lower resistance, indicating higher arousal, is associated with more rapid learning (Brown, 1937). The ends of the list were, as is usually found, learned more rapidly than the middle, and skin resistance was lower when the ends of the list were being presented. This finding provides an interesting line of evidence which is not usually taken into account when discussing reasons for the quicker learning of the ends of a list.

Several studies have shown that raising the level of activation during learning can improve long-term recall greatly, but leaves immediate recall either unaffected or actually impaired (Walker & Tarte, 1963; Kleinsmith & Kaplan, 1963, 1964; Berlyne et al., 1966; Batten, 1967). The improvement of long-term recall is presumably due to activation facilitating long-term registration and thus reducing the rate of forgetting. Why activation facilitates this registration is not clear, but a moderate level of activation would probably strengthen the signals entering the long-term memory store and perhaps strengthen those already there. Russell (1959) has put forward the interesting idea that random or rhythmic activity in the brain will tend to channel through established pathways and to confirm them; thus, if memory traces can be conceived as pathways, they will be strengthened. The impairment of immediate recall is presumably due to the muscle tension, noise, or other activating agent used during learning. These activating agents tend to produce neural noise which takes some time to die away and, until it has done so, is likely to confuse recall.

Associations with emotion

Current interest in activation and arousal seems to have come largely from Lindsley's (1951) suggestion that the excited emotions of fear and anger can be thought of as states of heightened arousal. Such a view provides, in terms of the model proposed here, a solution of the long-standing controversy about whether emotions "organize" or "disorganize" performance. Mild degrees of emotion, producing moderate degrees of arousal, are likely to be beneficial and therefore "organizing"; more severe degrees will lead to disruption of performance and thus be "disorganizing." This view tallies well with the observations made by Mira (1944) of fear reactions to civilian bombing during the Spanish Civil War. Mild degrees of fear, he suggested, led to prudence, self-restraint, concentration, and caution, and tended to improve achievement. More severe degrees of fear led to anxiety and alarm accompanied by breakdown of high-grade skills, disorganized activity, and tremors. Very severe degrees of fear resulted in panic marked by uncontrolled activity and loss of memory afterwards of what had happened, or in extreme cases led to collapse into a kind of tense stupor. Such extreme states would be likely to result if the stream of diffuse impulses from the brain stem became so intense that the cells of the cortex were not merely rendered more sensitive, but were actually fired. This would lead to many ill-organized, conflicting actions being initiated together. The cortex would be virtually inoperative in any significant way, and would justify Darrow's (1935) description of strong emotions as states of "relative functional decortication," similar to those produced in animals whose cortices have been surgically removed.

Stress and difficulty of task

Several studies of discrimination have found that performance improves with increase of reward for correct response, or with punishment for error. This improvement continues up to a certain point, but thereafter declines. Studies have further shown that the optimum level is lower for difficult than for easy tasks. The classical studies along these lines are those of Yerkes and Dodson (1908) and the effect is known as the *Yerkes-Dodson law.* It is reasonable to link these studies with those of stress, assuming that incentives, whether in the form of rewards or of punishments, tend to raise the level of arousal. If so, the Yerkes-Dodson law follows directly from the model we have postulated. Let us consider the case in which one of two possible quantities is presented at a time and the subject must say which is the greater or the lesser. The two quantities can be thought of as forming the two distributions in Figures 2.1 and 2.2, which will be closer together in a difficult task, where the quantities are closely similar, than in an easy task in which the quantities differ greatly. The three curves in Figure 7.3 are for three levels of difference. It can be seen that as the difference becomes greater, maximum performance rises and the optimum occurs at a higher level of arousal.

If the quantities to be discriminated were presented together instead of one at a time, the relationship between difficulty of task, point of maximum performance, and level of arousal would differ according to the way in which subjects made their judgments. For example, in Yerkes and Dodson's original experiment, the task was to choose the lighter of two grays presented side by side. The relationships in Figures 7.2 and 7.3 would hold if the subject either made an absolute judgment that, say, the right hand gray was the lighter or darker of the two shades, or judged that it was "light" or "dark" in relation to the left hand gray, or to some average of both. The model would still hold if the subject judged sometimes in terms of the right hand gray and sometimes of the left. If the subject judged in terms of the *differences* between the two stimuli in the way suggested by Vickers (1970) and outlined in Chapter 2, maximum performance would appear to be attained at *lower* arousal levels for easy than for difficult discriminations. However, as arousal rose beyond optimum, performance of easy tasks would remain high for much longer than that of difficult tasks. Also, the maximum performance with easy tasks at low arousal levels might not be attained, because at these levels the making of responses to signify the discriminations might become unreliable. Overall, therefore, performance would probably not differ greatly from that indicated in Figure 7.3.

Three further points may be made briefly. First, the scheme envisaged in Figures 7.2 and 7.3 would apply only if it is indeed true that increased arousal brings about a roughly proportionate increase of both signal and noise, leaving the ratio between them relatively little changed. It seems possible that in some cases this might not hold, but that noise would increase more than signal. This would be likely at very high levels of arousal since the system would tend to become so active due to noise alone that little extra activity would be possible when signals arrived. Such a disproportionate increase of noise would impair performance more with difficult discriminations than with easy ones, and thus enhance the effect shown in Figure 7.3. Experimental evidence has been obtained by Nettelbeck (1972), who found that noise in a discrimination task, measured in the manner described in Chapter 2, increased substantially when the subject was given electric shocks at random intervals during the session.

Second, changes of reward for correct responses and of punishment for errors affect the probable gains and risks attached to different responses and are therefore likely to alter the placing of the cutoff. Raising the cutoff level would have the effect of shifting the curves in Figure 7.3 to the right, and of exaggerating the separation between the curves for different levels of difficulty.

Third, we noted in Chapter 6 that if nerve impulses pass a synapse repeatedly its resistance is lowered so that it is more easily passed by further impulses on subsequent occasions (Eccles, 1953). This principle has been the basis of some influential theories of learning (e.g., Hebb, 1949). These theories hold that material to be learned produces a pattern of neural activity which is preserved as a pattern of lowered synaptic resistances. If this is true, it appears to follow that the unpatterned neural activity associated with high levels of stress would tend to produce widespread random lowering of synaptic resistances. In a moderate degree, this would merely sensitize a brain that would otherwise be relatively inert. However, prolonged severe stress might result in a breakdown of the normal "insulation" of one cell from another and thus lead to blurring of patterned brain activity. The effect would be more serious with difficult than with easy tasks since the signal-to-noise ratio would be lower in difficult tasks, and thus the effects of any blurring would be greater.

Individual differences in stress and motivation effects

Individuals differ greatly in their capacities and in the demands made upon them by circumstances and by their own aims. It is thus not surprising that they differ also in their reactions to stressful conditions. Recent discussion has particularly concentrated, however, on two broad variations: first, the extent to which arousal level rises with positive stress and, second, the chronic level of arousal (see e.g., Welford, 1965, 1968).

The first type of variation, between extremes of stability and instability, has been linked to Eysenck's (1965, 1970) concept of neuroticism and to Taylor's (1953) measure of anxiety. The second type, chronic level of arousal, appears to be related to Eysenck's dimension of extraversion-introversion; introversion, somewhat surprisingly, represents greater chronic arousal levels than extraversion. Research has concentrated mainly on this second relationship, and there is now an impressive array of evidence linking personality scores, autonomic indications of arousal, and performance.

Due to the greater arousal of more introverted subjects compared with those more extraverted, introverts tend to be better performers under monotonous conditions where arousal tends to sag, to be less affected by narcotic drugs, to stand up better to loss of sleep, and to have fewer traffic accidents— presumably because they are more alert (Fine, 1963). Also, the diurnal rise and fall of body temperature occurs earlier in the day in introverts, so that they are warmer and perform better than extraverts in the morning, although the latter tend to catch up during the afternoon (Colquhoun, 1960; Colquhoun & Corcoran, 1964; Blake, 1967).

Nettelbeck (1973b), who examined the relationships between personality test scores and the various measures in the discrimination task outlined in Chapter 2, found that introverts tended to make more use of stored information than extraverts. He also found that those who obtained extremely high scores for either extraversion, introversion, stability or instability, or extremely low scores for anxiety tended to have longer inspection times than those with more moderate scores. It is understandable that this might characterize those with extremely high scores for extraversion or stability and extremely low scores for anxiety, because these people tend to be relatively inert. The reason why those with extreme scores for introversion and instability have long inspection times is, however, not so obvious. Nettelbeck suggested that longer times might be a means of offsetting increased noise in these subjects: he pointed out that because of their high arousal levels, they might otherwise have been expected to show much higher noise levels than in fact they did.

The personality variables of introversion and extraversion and their seeming basis in differences of arousability and chronic arousal level appear to have widespread ramifications. For example, in everyday life, introverts tend to seek peace and quiet, to prefer subdued colors, and to be generally sensitive and restrained. They tend to be self-driving and, as one would expect from the inverted-U relationship of Figure 7.1, make the best use of their powers if not driven hard. Extraverts, on the contrary, tend to enjoy noise, bright colors, and seem actively to seek stimulation, as if without it they would be less than optimally aroused. As would again be expected from Figure 7.1, extraverts tend to remain stable under pressure and to perform best under such conditions.

An illustration of these distinctions between the introvert and the extravert is contained in the contrast between two studies relating personality to examination performance by students. Furneaux (1962) reported a study of first-year engineering students at a British university, in which he found that the best examination performances at the end of the year were by those whose personalities tended towards both instability and introversion. The worst performances were by those at the opposite ends of both these dimensions, that is, the stable extraverts. The study was repeated on students in an Australian college of advanced education with diametrically opposite results: the stable extraverts did best, and the unstable introverts worst (Killingsworth, 1972). It is not certain why the results of the two studies should have differed, but it seems fairly clear that at least part of the reason is that the students in the second study had been driven harder in their courses than those in the first. Whatever the reasons, the results suggest that both institutions were wasting, or failing to recognize, some of their best talent. It seems likely that many failures in each school could have been avoided if the pressures put on individual students had been adjusted to their personalities.

Some of the differences between extraverts and introverts seem to be mirrored in certain forms of mental handicap. Thus many retardates show extravert characteristics and many psychiatric cases show introvert. In these individuals, extraversion and introversion both tend to be exaggerated, plausibly reflecting extreme differences of chronic arousal level. This has some important implications for the employment of handicapped persons. For example, many retardates seem to tolerate noisy, socially stimulating conditions better than psychiatric cases (McEwen, 1973).

Other individual differences of motivation and stress seen both in the laboratory and in real life can reasonably be ascribed to differences in the functioning of the main chain of mechanisms implied in the system outlined in Chapter 1. An example of the effects of failure to comprehend incoming data can be seen in the way in which many old people whose interests have been reduced to their own ailments and past achievements fail to communicate with others and become listless and apathetic. Individual differences in the way signals are translated into action can be seen in the range of human interest from things to people, from words to numbers, from ideas to action—all seem to reflect skills in dealing with different materials and situations.

Some of the most important individual differences seem to lie in the observation of feedback. For instance, it is probably true that job satisfaction, morale, enthusiasm, and willingness to expend effort depend largely on being able to feel that one can make a significant contribution to the effectiveness of the organization in which one works. In a different sphere, an essential shortcoming of many delinquents and criminals appears to lie in their inability to recognize the ways in which their actions affect their environment and other people in it. Their behavior is thus relatively uncontrolled, and needs to be extreme if it is to have what are, to them, observable and satisfying effects.

A further important way in which individuals differ seems to be in the extent to which immediate desires can be set aside in favor of long-term aims. Several studies have linked this ability to factors of childhood training, and to social variables such as occupational class (for a review see Welford, 1971a). Ability to work for distant goals is perhaps epitomized in a simple way by the capacities to delay action and to work for deferred rewards, and may contain a deep-seated biological foundation in that these capacities tend to increase as one goes up the mammalian evolutionary scale.

While the relationship of these individual differences to other variables is fairly clear, the direction of cause and effect is often uncertain. Is failure to observe the reactions of others a cause of delinquency, or does the delinquent direct attention away from others? Is the ability to pursue long-term aims fostered by middle-class conditions, or is it a trait which tends to bring individuals into the middle class and keep them there? Are reactivity to stress and chronic arousal level innately determined personality characteristics, or do they reflect the extent of exposure to stress in earlier life? At present, we cannot answer these questions.

Perhaps the truth is to be found in the two-way cumulative relationship suggested earlier, in which capacity develops from aim and aim from capacity. If so, it has important implications for the perennial problem of "nature" and "nurture" as factors to be taken into account in understanding human behavior and framing social policies. Obviously, the person who is concerned to make the world a better place must proceed as if the influences were from the environment towards the individual. Doing so blindly and uncritically, however, is likely to lead at best to a great deal of wasted effort and disappointment, and at worst to serious errors of policy. It cannot be assumed that production of a uniformly good environment will ensure everyone's happiness and well-being. There must instead be a more complex, detailed matching of environments to people, recognizing that individuals differ and that their various interests, desires, needs, and aims cannot be flattened into uniformity without giving rise to serious stresses due to frustration.

Fatigue

The deterioration of performance when a stressful task is continued for a long time has traditionally been attributed to fatigue, conceived of as some kind of impairment in one or more of the brain and body mechanisms involved. The concept of fatigue comes from studies of muscular performance: if a muscle is exercised continuously at a rapid rate, the strength of its contraction gradually falls until it ceases altogether. After a short rest, strength of contraction is partially restored, and after a longer rest, is fully restored. Fundamentally, the loss of performance is due to lack of oxygen and the accumulation of waste products in the muscle. However, two facts indicate that central mechanisms are also involved.

First, contraction usually ceases because the nerve impulses stimulating the muscle have ceased—it can still be made to contract by direct electrical stimulation. The nerve impulses appear to fail because some feedback to the brain signals that an overload has occurred, and the failure can be regarded as a reaction designed to protect the overloaded muscle and the bones to which it is attached. On the conscious level, this feedback often appears as pain, and contraction ceases when the pain exceeds the level the subject is willing to tolerate. A failure of motivation results, but motivation can be extended by suitable incentives. A striking illustration is given by Schwab (1953), who required subjects to hang from a horizontal bar. He found that with instructions to hold on "as long as possible," the average length of time before letting go was less than 1 minute. With strong urging, the hanging time was somewhat increased. When a $5 reward was promised for bettering their previous records, subjects managed to hang on for an average of nearly 2 minutes.

Second, as contraction in one muscle begins to fail, other muscles become active in a manner which suggests an unconscious attempt to relieve the fatiguing muscle by shifting its load to other muscles. This *recruitment* begins with muscles close to the one that is tiring, but gradually spreads to more remote muscles.

It has traditionally been assumed that states of "mental fatigue" which are analogous to those of muscular fatigue can be identified. For the analogy to hold, mental fatigue must imply the impairment of some brain mechanism as a result of long-continued use. The impairment must be reversible in the sense that it disappears with rest, and may take the form of lowered sensitivity, responsiveness, or capacity. Lowered capacity may be seen as a reduction in either the amount of information that can be handled at any one instant, and thus in reduced "mental power," or in the amount of information that can be handled in a given period, and so in slowness of perception, choice, and so on.

Impairments of performance which may be attributable to mental fatigue can be summarized under five headings: perceptual changes, slowing of performance, irregularity of timing, disorganization of performance, and temporary improvement of performance.

Perceptual changes

Several studies have shown that visual acuity and critical flicker frequency (CFF) decrease in the course of repeated measurements taken continuously over periods of half an hour or so (e.g., Berger & Mahneke, 1954). These decreases cannot be attributed to reduction of pupil size (Grandjean & Perret, 1961). At a more complex level, Saldanha (1955, 1957) found that repeated settings made on the vernier scale of a caliper gauge for half an hour or more became less regular, and thus less accurate, with time, but that accuracy returned after about half an hour of rest. We may note in passing that the return was greater after a period of rest than after a similar period spent canceling Landolt rings (incomplete rings or circles used in studying visual acuity)—the fatigue effect was such that a change of work was not as good as a rest. The motor components in all these tasks were trivial, and thus it is clear that there was some loss of fine differentiation either spatially, as with visual acuity or vernier settings, or temporally as with CFF.

CFF and its auditory counterpart, critical flutter frequency—the frequency at which an intermittent tone comes to appear continuous—also decrease after mental work such as calculating, reading, or problem-solving (Simonson & Brozek, 1952; Davis, 1955; Grandjean & Perret, 1961). When considering the mechanism involved, it should be noted that CFF has also been found to decrease following brain injury and under the influence of depressant drugs, and to decrease progressively with age during adulthood, a time when there is a continual loss of active brain cells.

Slowing of performance

One of the most frequently observed effects of fatigue is the slowing of sensory-motor performance. This may be due to muscular fatigue, but there is no doubt that central mechanism factors are often, and probably mainly, involved. An indication of this is contained in the results of an experiment by Singleton (1953) who used a serial choice-reaction task. He found that performance became slower during a run, but that this was due to slowing of reaction times rather than movement times—that is, in deciding what movement to make rather than in executing it. The degree of slowing increased as the compatibility of the signals and actions fell, or, in other words, as the central demands of the task rose.

Slowness may cause several complications when the subject cannot, as in Singleton's case, work at his own pace, but is externally paced or under severe pressure for speed. In particular, some of the actions required may be omitted, especially responses to signals which are ancillary to the main task or on the periphery of the display (Davis, 1948; Bursill, 1958). Such omissions may be regarded as spontaneous attempts to simplify the task. Alternatively, the subject may try to complete all the actions required and will in consequence hurry and make errors. In these circumstances, a vicious circle situation can easily develop: the subject hurries and makes an error, correcting the error delays him so that he hurries even more and makes more errors, and so on.

Irregularity of timing

Long-continued performance tends to become not only slower but also less regular. Striking illustrations of these tendencies have come from industrial tasks in which, during a shift, a moderate rise has occurred in the mean time required to perform each cycle of an operation, accompanied by a much greater rise in the standard deviation (for a review see Murrell, 1965). To some extent, irregularity may be more apparent than real. The distributions of times for individual cycles of repetitive tasks tend to be skewed, with a tail of very long times and with a variance increasing with the mean; any overall slowing will therefore increase the variance and the number of what seem to be unusually long times. An alternate explanation (Bills, 1931) suggests that irregularity of performance is due to occasional "blocking." That is, every now and then a short gap appears in an otherwise rapid performance, and the frequency of such gaps increases when the task is continued for a long time.

Clear evidence of such blocking was obtained in a serial reaction task by Bertelson and Joffe (1963). Looking at the distributions of the reaction times during runs of 30 minutes, they found no change in the averages of the shorter or the median reaction times, but a marked increase in the average of the longer reaction times. The percentage of "blocks" (defined as reaction times longer than twice the mean) rose rapidly during the first 5 minutes of work and slowly thereafter. More important, there was a tendency for reaction times and errors to rise during the responses immediately before a block, and to fall immediately after. The results are consistent with the view that some kind of fatigue effect builds up gradually over a series of responses which is dissipated by the block. It should be noted that according to this view, there are two fatigue effects involved: a short-term effect dissipated at each block, and a longer-term effect which causes a rise in the frequency of blocks. The longer-term effect might be due to incomplete recovery during a block, so that the time taken to build up to the next block is shorter than it would otherwise have been.

Disorganization of performance

Fatigued subjects sometimes perform correct actions, but in the wrong order. In other words, the coordination of their performance, the ordering of individual actions into "larger units," has broken down (Bartlett, 1943). This line of thought has not been followed up to the extent it deserves, probably because it is not easy to study the kinds of complex performance in which such breakdowns might occur. It does, however, tally well with the mild confusion, inability for sustained thought, and impairment of judgment often observed in states of fatigue. Two possible factors seem to justify further research:

1. *Impairment of routine.* When a situation or task is encountered repeatedly, we tend spontaneously, as discussed in Chapter 5, to build routines that enable us to treat several actions together as a single ordered "unit," instead of having to make individual decisions about each one. The building of such units depends, however, upon the ability to carry out the individual actions accurately enough for one to follow another without the flow having to be interrupted in order to make corrections. Any change due to fatigue or any other factor that impairs accuracy will tend to break up these routines and make it necessary once more to deal with the task piecemeal.

2. *Disturbance of short-term retention.* We have noted in previous chapters that implicit in the concept of organized performance and the integration of actions or information is some form of short-term retention that holds earlier items to be combined with later ones and keeps a tally of what has been done and what remains to be done. Such short-term retention is very susceptible to disruption by shifts of attention, especially after brain injury, in old age, and with other conditions in which some organic impairment can be presumed. There is some evidence of a similar breakdown with fatigue from tests on civilian aircrews. In one experiment (Welford, Brown, & Gabb, 1950), radio officers were tested with a type of electrical problem before and after flights from the United Kingdom to Africa, India, Australia, or the Far East. Subjects were given a box with six terminals on the top, a circuit diagram, and a resistance meter and had to determine which terminal on the box corresponded to each on the diagram by taking readings on the meter. Subjects made many more readings if they took the test after a flight than before, and it was clear that while taking one reading they were forgetting others already obtained, and so had to take some readings several times.

Temporary improvement of performance

Somewhat surprisingly, the first sign of oncoming fatigue is sometimes an improvement of performance, in the sense that performance becomes more active and achievement rises; deterioration does not set in until later. For example, in another experiment on the radio officers who took part in the electrical problem experiment, performance at a plotting task was better after a flight with a relatively easy schedule than it was before going out. Performance was, however, poorer after a trip with a more arduous schedule than it was before flight, and the improved performance after an easy trip occurred only with the relatively easy plotting task; it did not occur with the more difficult electrical problems.

Explanations of mental fatigue

Two main lines of explanation have been offered for mental fatigue. The traditional assumption is that some group of nerve cells concerned with the fatiguing performance, or with some essential link in it, becomes insensitive or unresponsive through continued activity. Such a view explains well the similarity of some fatigue effects, such as a decrease of CFF, to those of brain injury. It can account for slowing of performance by assuming that some stage in the sensory-motor chain requires a stronger stimulus to operate it and that stimulation can be integrated over time. Blocking is accounted for by assuming that the breakdown may be of only short duration. Loss of short-term retention would result if the self-maintaining neuronal circuits, on which it must almost certainly depend, became insensitive, so allowing the memory traces to decay.

Rest, according to this view, permits recovery of the nerve cells involved. Overactivity and improved performance in the early stages of fatigue can be accounted for either by analogy with the recruitment effect found in neuromuscular fatigue or by assuming that, faced with incipient failure, the subject makes compensatory increases of effort that may, for a time, more than offset losses due to fatigue.

The alternative type of explanation regards fatigue as an overarousal effect (Bartley & Chute, 1947; Woodworth & Schlosberg, 1954; Crawford, 1961). In this case, fatigue results when neural activity, either general or local, rises beyond some optimum level. Such a theory accounts for sensory fatigue directly in terms of the blurring effects of neural noise. It accounts for slowing of performance by arguing that the effective strength of stimuli from one part of the sensory-motor mechanism to another should be measured in terms of signal-to-noise ratio, and that a rise in the noise level thus implies a need for more powerful signals in order to maintain the ratio required. Increased neural noise, leading to brief periods of specially intense neural activity, could account for blocking and for brief periods during which unwanted signals or responses might be facilitated and cause distraction. Loss of short-term retention is assumed to result from disturbance rather than decay of the memory traces. Rest allows excess activity or sensitivity to die away. Overactivity and improved performance during the early stages of fatigue are accounted for directly by facilitatory effects of mild rises in arousal.

Present data on fatigue seem to be equivocal in the sense that they are consistent, given plausible supplementary hypotheses, with either view. Indeed, the two processes may well both operate in different circumstances. Some indications in favor of the arousal theory are perhaps contained in the irritability and difficulty of relaxing or sleeping often observed after a long period of taxing mental work, and in the finding that a focusing of attention similar to that found in states regarded as fatiguing also occurs in the presence of loud noise which is regarded as arousing (Hamilton & Copeman, 1970; Hockey, 1970a, b).

On the other hand, Berger and Mahneke's (1954) results suggest impairment when the effects of the two mechanisms are compared in terms of signal-detection theory. Local neural failure would be expected to reduce d', whereas overarousal would be expected to lower β. Moderate overarousal would leave d' little changed, but if overarousal was so intense that cells in the cortex were not merely sensitized but actually fired, the increased noise that would result might lower d' as well as β. Berger and Mahneke's results have been interpreted as implying a fall of d' without a change of β (Mackworth & Taylor, 1963).

Vigilance

The extensive experimental work on the maintenance of vigilance undertaken since World War II arose from the fact that, when radar operators and lookouts watch for infrequent signals, they tend to miss these signals after they have been on watch for an hour or so. Research in this area has gained attention not only because of its interest to the military, but for its obvious implications for inspection and monitoring work in industry and because it raises important theoretical issues as well.

Initial experiments on simulated radar displays and other laboratory tasks made it clear that the proportion of signals detected fell sharply over a period of half an hour or so when the signals were faint, brief, and infrequent. With radar-type displays showing signals at unpredictable intervals, it could be argued that the subjects, in order to be sure of seeing them when they occurred, had to make a rapid and continuous series of checks. These could be fatiguing, and the fall in performance might therefore be a fatigue effect. Other laboratory tasks, however, have presented subjects with clearly observable signals at discrete intervals and required them to detect occasional signals slightly different from the majority. In these tasks, the intervals were too long (1 to 5 seconds) to make a fatigue theory tenable; some other factor is clearly involved (for reviews see Broadbent, 1958, 1971; Mackworth, 1969, 1970; Davies & Tune, 1970).

The theory which most adequately explains the main facts obtained in what is now a vast array of experiments is that the monotonous conditions of vigilance tasks cause the level of arousal to fall. Evidence for this view comes from the fact that various indices of autonomic activity decrease as vigilance falls (e.g., Nishioka et al., 1960; Dardano, 1962; Eason et al., 1965). Also, vigilance does not deteriorate under conditions likely to stimulate the diffuse activating system, such as when knowledge of results is provided (e.g., Wilkinson, 1964), or when subjects are given benzedrine, a drug known to increase arousal (Mackworth, 1950). Further, vigilance is improved by any brief change in conditions during a watch, such as receiving a telephone call (Mackworth, 1950). This last result is perhaps paralleled by the finding in industry that output may increase if workers change from one job to another during a shift (Vernon, 1924; Wyatt & Langdon, 1932). At the same time, decision criteria may shift as predicted by Equation 2.8.

If this theory is correct, we should expect that during a monotonous watch conditions of detection would change from those of Figure 7.2B to those of Figure 7.2A, and that β would rise while d' would be little changed. Several experiments have shown this to occur (e.g., Broadbent & Gregory, 1963; Loeb & Binford, 1964). Subjectively, the change would appear as a decrease in motivation or as an expectation that nothing was likely to occur. Objectively, it might appear as momentary lapses of attention. These lapses would be most serious when signals were brief; signals of longer duration might not be missed but, instead, might be reacted to more slowly, because of having to wait until the lapse was over to secure attention. Figure 7.2 also implies that the effects would be less serious if the signals were stronger, since the distributions for noise and signal would be farther apart and more of the latter would be likely to fall above the cutoff. All these points have been verified by experimental evidence.

A few findings which do not fit the general trend can perhaps be regarded as due to the fact that the tasks concerned were fatiguing as well as monotonous. For example, experiments in which subjects had to detect momentary interruptions in the movement of a pointer rotating continuously round a dial showed that d' fell substantially with time (Mackworth & Taylor, 1963; Mackworth, 1964, 1965). The significant feature of this task was that signals might occur at any time instead of at discrete intervals. Watching had to be absolutely continuous or signals would be missed. Such a task is likely to be fatiguing indeed. The results of these experiments are interesting since they point to a possible means of distinguishing between the effects of fatigue and monotony. We have already noted that fatigue effects should lead to a *fall* of either d', β, or both. Monotony in the absence of fatigue should always, if it has any effect, lead to a *rise* of β with little or no change of d'.

Effects of skill on the performance of stressful, fatiguing, and monotonous tasks

We have already noted some ways in which the exercise of skill reduces susceptibility to stress, fatigue, and monotony. Five additional ways follow from what has been said in previous chapters:

(a) The perceptual coding mentioned in Chapter 3, and the response coding and motor sequencing discussed in Chapters 4 and 5, have the effect of enabling the subject to deal with the task in larger units. A person can thus operate effectively with fewer decisions in a given period of time. Since pressure for speed is one of the most powerful causes of stress and fatigue, coding and sequencing can effectively reduce them. Coding and sequencing can perhaps also improve vigilance in monotonous conditions, in that the larger units might be more varied than the detailed smaller units of which they were made up. For instance, a meaningless series of dots and dashes would be more monotonous than a message in Morse code where patterns of dots and dashes could be interpreted as letters and words.

(b) Coding of incoming sequences makes it possible to predict when and where significant events are likely to occur, and thus to direct attention efficiently. This is another means to economy of decision, and thus to reduction of stress and fatigue. Coding of incoming sequences is also likely to improve vigilance since it enables attention to be concentrated at appropriate places and times. However, the imposition of a code which is only approximately correct can lead to incorrect expectations which divert attention from where it is needed. An example is provided by the engineer of a train who passed a red signal when he was expecting green because, as he said, "I have never been stopped there in the whole time I have been traveling" (Davis, 1958, 1966).

(c) The increased accuracy of ballistic actions that comes with long practice also tends to reduce stress and fatigue, by lessening the time and effort required to correct errors and to monitor action. Increased accuracy is also likely to reduce the stress resulting from anxiety, which seems typically to arise from anticipation of failure.

(d) A skill specifically aimed at avoiding stress and fatigue lies in pacing performance so that it always remains within one's capacity. In the case of muscular work, such as that involved in long-distance running or cycling, the importance of such pacing is well recognized (e.g., Ward, 1950). Pacing essentially ensures that energy output does not exceed the capacity of the cardiovascular system to replace oxygen and remove waste products of muscle action while exertion is required. To what extent muscular and mental performances are comparable in this regard is not clear, but it seems reasonable to suppose that a balance could be struck between the rates at which any local neural failure might build up and recover, and between the increase and dissipation of overarousal. An analogous balance could, perhaps, be struck between tendencies to underarousal and efforts to restore optimum. Certainly people can by an effort of will sometimes postpone states of underarousal, as evidenced by the ability to maintain attention even when bored, or to remain awake when desiring to sleep.

(e) Perhaps the most pervasive means of avoiding all the adverse effects discussed in this chapter lies in the subtle and little recognized skill of matching aims and ambitions realistically to capacities and opportunities. In this way it is possible to avoid the extremes, both of the thrusting drive associated with heart disease and many other symptoms of stress, and of the idleness which, however attractive in prospect, quickly becomes monotonous and boring in actuality. The time seems to have come when knowledge of human skill could provide a more precise and factual understanding of these extremes.

Summary

Motivation arises when there is some departure from optimum in the state of the organism, and results in action which attempts to restore optimum conditions. Stress arises when the action fails to restore the optimum state. This simple scheme can account for many facts of both motivation and stress, and also of emotion. However, to cover anything like the full range of facts, four additional principles need to be added:

(a) Action may be attempted in anticipation of a departure from optimum.
(b) Willingness to undertake action appears to depend upon the extent to which the benefits likely to result are offset by the cost, effort, or unpleasantness of obtaining them.
(c) Normally any one action results from a whole hierarchy of motives on different time scales, the longer term tending to control and organize the shorter term.
(d) Optimum states imply moderate degrees of stimulation, variety or predictability, and conflict. Departures from optimum may be either in the direction of excess or insufficiency. These variables can be regarded as affecting arousal, so that optimum can be defined in terms of a moderate degree of arousal.

Peak levels in various types of performance, learning, and memory are reached at moderate levels of arousal. The reason can be inferred in terms of signal detection theory: underarousal leads to a rise of β so that many signals are missed, whereas overarousal leads to a fall of β and an increase in false positives. The theory predicts that the level of arousal at which performance is optimum is lower for more difficult tasks, in conformity with the Yerkes-Dodson law.

Many individual differences of motivation can be attributed to differences of either arousability when departure from optimum occurs, or of normal chronic arousal level. The former seems to be associated with instability-stability and the latter with introversion-extraversion. Some other individual differences of motivation appear to be due to differences in the functioning of the main chain of information processing mechanisms, and in the ability to set aside short-term for longer-term motives.

There appear to be important motivational factors in muscular fatigue. How far mental and muscular fatigue are analogous is questionable. The main phenomena of mental fatigue can be seen as:

(a) Certain perceptual changes, for example in visual acuity and critical flicker frequency.
(b) Slowing of performance, sometimes partly compensated for by restriction of attention or other attempts to reduce load.
(c) Irregularity in the timing of action, and intermittent "blocking."
(d) Disorganization of action, seemingly due to disruption of routines and impairment of short-term retention.
(e) With easy tasks, the effects of mild degrees of fatigue may be a temporary improvement of performance.

The two main explanations that have been offered of mental fatigue are in terms of, first, temporary local neural failure in one or another of the brain mechanisms; and second, overarousal. Both theories can account for most of the facts known so far.

The loss of vigilance seen in monotonous tasks appears to be the result of underarousal, leading to a rise of β. It is thus to be distinguished from fatigue which would be expected to lead to a fall of either β or d' or both. The evidence is confused by the fact that some tasks are both monotonous and fatiguing.

Skill in avoiding the adverse effects of stress, fatigue, and monotony is shown in various ways including:

(a) More thorough coding of perception and action which enables tasks to be done with fewer but more varied decisions.
(b) Prediction of events and deployment of attention to meet them. This has, however, the attendant danger that false expectations may divert attention from where it is needed.
(c) Pacing of performance so as to avoid periods of over- or underloading.
(d) Realistic ordering of aims.

Social skill

8

Studies of sensory-motor skill have typically been of people operating machines, whether in industry or the military or the laboratory. The performance of man and machine together has essentially depended on the characteristics of both, and on their interaction in what has come to be termed a *system* (see Singleton et al., 1967). It seems fair to argue that there is a close analogy between such man-machine systems and social groups whose members are in communication with one another, and that knowledge we possess of the first could help in understanding the second—indeed, is fundamental to it.

An operator manipulates the controls of a machine which responds by adjusting its operation in accordance with their setting. The machine gives rise to output and to indications on meters or other signaling devices which the operator observes, thus closing the feedback loop. If we regard the controls as the machine's perceptual system and its output and signaling devices as its effectors, there is a close analogy of machine operation with conversation between person and person. One person speaks or takes some action which another individual observes and uses as the basis of responding action. In turn, the first person observes the response and uses it to shape his or her own subsequent action, and so on. Just as skill in operating a machine consists of interpreting its indications and controlling it to obtain the desired output, so interpersonal skill consists essentially of interpreting and controlling the communications coming from another person, and in designing one's own communications to produce desired reactions.

Let us consider this human interaction in terms of the main information flow set out in Figure 1.1.

Coding of perception and action in social situations

Social communication obviously depends upon each of the parties concerned being able to understand the other. It is therefore easier when they share the same language, and this is true not only in the sense of verbal language, but also includes the nonverbal signs and nuances by which a great deal of information is conveyed (Argyle, 1967).

However, skill in conveying information to others and interpreting it from them does not depend only on language whether of word or gesture. It depends also on the messages to be conveyed being couched in terms of the interests, attitudes, and codings of experience by the other person and thus depends upon knowledge of the other person. Messages must also be appropriate to the situation of the moment, so that it is often necessary to select times and places if they are to be accepted. Furthermore, some kinds of presentation may overload the receiver. This is so not only when the speaker conveys ideas too fast, but when the ideas are arranged or delivered in such a way as to make severe demands upon short-term retention. Consider, for example, the following statement:

> "You're just the person I wanted to see to ask a question! I was walking along Main Street last Tuesday—no, wait a minute, was it Tuesday or Wednesday? Let me see, I had my hair done on Tuesday afternoon and it must have been after that because just before I met Uncle George I ran into that woman with the lisp who lives down the street and she said, 'Your hair lookth tho lovely,' and I said, 'Thank you very much, I always have it done at Martha's because the girls are so nice there.' Well, never mind which day it was, Uncle George—he was my father's brother who lived for a long time in Singapore and still has two sons living there, such charming boys, one is in a shipping office, I can't remember the company, and the other runs a hotel, I think; of course I haven't met their wives, but the one in the shipping office has three children, two girls and a boy, and the other has two—one of each. I've got photographs of them right here in my bag, I think, and I'm sure you'll agree they are really delightful, and they often write to their old cousin even though they have never seen her. He asked me if I would have dinner with him on Saturday, and of course I said I would, he is so charming and his daughter is such a wonderful cook—you should just try her apricot soufflé, it is really out of this world. And he said, 'Do you know anyone else who would like to come and make it a foursome,' so naturally, I thought of you."

The essential information that the speaker's Uncle George is extending an invitation for dinner on Saturday is embedded in a mass of irrelevant matter, but there is no indication of what is relevant and what is not until the end, so that all the information conveyed must be retained until then. We may note that this kind of overload is found also in other types of communication. For example, the commonly preferred method of writing scientific papers is to outline the problem in an introduction, then describe the methods for a series of experiments, then list all the results of the series, and only then interpret them and discuss their significance. The reader has to retain all the details of introduction, methods, and results in order to understand the discussion at the end. What is, from the reader's point of view, a much easier alternative is to describe the method and results for one experiment at a time, and to interpret and discuss each result before passing on to the next.

As regards the receiver, one can observe social techniques which reflect various points made in earlier chapters. One trivial example is the repetition of the name of someone to whom one has been introduced—a procedure likely to help its registration in long-term memory. More interesting is the fact that some people are clearly more skilled than others at selecting and ordering material presented to them, and at retaining essentials while discarding what is irrelevant. This ability often seems to be well developed in lawyers and patent agents, who can listen to a client and then produce a statement which explains a position or an invention far more concisely and pertinently than the client can. What are the essentials of such skill and how it can be acquired are not known, but it appears not only to involve good short-term retention, but a capacity for rapid integration of data and choice of codes in which to store it in long-term memory.

Effects of failure to communicate—the example of race relations

Failure to convey information will leave the other party with unresolved uncertainties which, as implied in the previous chapter, are likely to produce anxiety and stress, and to give opportunities for misunderstanding, distrust, and fear. Such failure seems to be one of the factors involved in various kinds of social disharmony. Let us consider, by way of example, the question of antipathy between members of different races living in close proximity. We obviously cannot deal with this problem in detail, but it seems fair to suggest that any average differences between races in language, capacities, interests, personality traits, or social customs will make communication difficult because the codings used by the races will differ. Lack of full communication and understanding will increase the likelihood of error in dealing with the other race, and this in turn may lead to fear and withdrawal. The problem will be particularly acute when there are actual conflicts of meaning: when, for instance, a style of dress implies one set of personal characteristics among one race, and another among the other; or when the same action is interpreted differently by different races, so that courses of action in the presence of the other race have to be chosen with extra care if they are not to be misunderstood.

If this view is correct, three implications follow which do, in fact, seem to hold true in a general sense. First, friction will arise most frequently where substantial numbers of two or more races are living together in the same cities or neighborhoods, so that they have to take account of one another at all times (e.g., Kawwa, 1968): occasional, isolated members of another race met for limited periods tend to excite curiosity and interest rather than enmity. Second, attempts to reduce the complications involved in living close to members of another race by means of partial segregation are likely to be unsuccessful; they will cut the races off from one another, so that the uncertainty inherent in the remaining contacts will be increased. Third, the easiest relationships seem likely to exist when members of different races understand each other's reactions thoroughly. This last implication suggests the need for a great deal of instruction and education to break down language barriers and to provide members of all races with accurate, sympathetic, and unsentimental knowledge about the customs, problems, hopes, and fears of the other races, in the hope of changing divisive modes of thought and action.

Bringing about changes of social thought and action is, however, far from easy. Social attitudes, norms, and customs represent codifications of insights and techniques which provide ready-made solutions to recurrent problems, avoiding complex ad hoc decisions. They thus make for efficiency in day-to-day living and, as we have noted in previous chapters, are likely to be used unless pressures are strong for change. Modifications of attitudes, norms, and customs do indeed occur, presumably in response to changing circumstances or fresh insights into methods of dealing with the problems of living, but there is usually a considerable time lag between needs becoming apparent and the changes required to meet them being made. The slowness of the process means that if pressure for change is maintained until change actually occurs, it may go too far and require a counterchange later, so that the system will oscillate. This is especially a danger if changes are sought quickly and urgently.

Rate of information flow

One of the most important factors limiting social interaction is the time taken to process data, which was discussed briefly in Chapter 1 and more fully in Chapter 4. At the level of individual contacts, this limitation means that it is often more exacting to listen than to talk. Listening is an externally paced task in the sense that information has to be accepted at a speed determined by the speaker, so that the listener is subject to risk of overload. Even if the speaker's average rate of presentation is within the listener's capacity, there are likely to be peaks at which a temporary overload will occur. Talking, in contrast, is done at a speed determined by the speaker, who can normally adjust the rate of output to suit his or her own capacities.

The time taken to process data is especially important in the communication systems of industries and other large organizations (Welford, 1966a). The communication charts often seen on the walls of those running such organizations give a very incomplete indication of the relevant features of the system. To obtain an adequate picture, it would be necessary to ask a range of detailed questions about each individual in the communication chain. What is the variety of decisions as well as the number of decisions to be made? How many sources of data have to be coordinated? How directly do the data received indicate the appropriate action to take? Are all the data for a given decision present at one time, or do some have to be carried in memory until other data arrive? Are the data clear and precise, or may they be unreliable or vacillating? Even if the average rate at which decisions have to be made is well within a person's capacity, are there periods of overload? How far can the individual differentiate the results of his or her actions from those of actions by others? The load on each individual in the chain can be viewed as one of conveying data from a display consisting of messages from other people, to responses in the form of various kinds of executive action, and can in principle be calculated in terms of Equation 4.4 (Leuba, 1967).

The concept of limited capacity to process data seems especially relevant to problems of leadership in relation to size of group. Harcourt (1959) suggested that the number of people one person can lead will depend on the amount of data requiring decision they generate: if they produce too much, the leader will be overloaded and will be liable to make hasty, ill-considered decisions. The amount of data individual members produce will depend on the nature of the job, the conditions under which it is done, and their personal characteristics. If they are performing a routine job under stable conditions and are of even temperament, one person will be able to lead a large number. If, however, the work is not of a routine nature and requires constant detailed attention, or if various members are doing different jobs, or if working conditions are unpredictable or there are unstable personalities among the team, the maximum size of group that one individual can lead effectively will be reduced.

When a group becomes too large for one person to lead, there seem to be two main alternative procedures available. First, members of the group can be required to refer particular problems to one of a range of specialists added to the group as deputy leaders. The disadvantage of this system is that individual members may have to make difficult decisions about which specialist to go to, and may find themselves having to try several before the right one to deal with their particular problem is found.

Alternatively, the group can be split into smaller subgroups, each with a leader who can call on specialists and is responsible in turn to a leader higher in a hierarchy. In this way the members are still able to refer all their problems to one person, and although the difficulty of getting the right specialist service may merely be transferred to the subgroup leader, the morale and effectiveness of the group as a whole is likely to be higher than if such decisions have to be made by individual members. The superiority of the second system is likely to increase with the frequency of problems requiring decisions for individual members. Thus, with a routine operation under stable conditions, there may be little to choose between the effectiveness of the two methods of organization, but if technical and management functions are highly complex, the second could be expected to yield better results.

Skill in avoiding overload can be seen at a relatively low level in attempts to reduce the flow of data from others. For example, a waiter in a restaurant may carefully avoid catching the eye of a diner at one table while he is serving those at another. Again, a politician in the news may be "not available for comment" until public interest has subsided. At an organizational level, skill consists of coding incoming data and devising routines of action which are simple in the sense of effectively covering the maximum number of contingencies with relatively few rules, leaving a minimum number of ad hoc decisions to be made.

Feedback

The model of social interaction presented here depends essentially upon the maintenance of feedback from each person involved to each other. When people get to know each other well, they may be able to predict the reactions of others accurately enough to act ballistically in larger units analogous to those discussed in Chapter 5. Some closure of the feedback loop is, however, still essential and social interaction will not continue for long if it is broken.

The need for feedback also has some important implications for industrial and other organizations. For example, an executive will be unable to dismiss a problem completely until some indication has been obtained of the effectiveness of any decision made, so that when assessing the executive's load it is necessary to ask how long it takes for such feedback to arrive. It is also pertinent to ask whether several feedbacks are received after different periods and, if so, whether the indications that come quickly differ from those that are slower—for example, does an action bring long-term benefits despite the fact that for a time it is unpopular with others working in the organization? Again, if a working group is to be adaptable to changing conditions, or is even to maintain a high standard in stable conditions, it must not only have clear instructions, but feedback of information about the quality of performance attained. This can be achieved to a limited extent by observation on the part of a foreman or manager of the end product of the group, but much fuller information will obviously be obtained when there is rapid and easy two-way communication between the manager and the managed which gives detailed insight into difficulties encountered and ideas about how they might be overcome. In stable conditions, once the methods for a job have been established, it is possible to run on satisfactorily for an appreciable time without such feedback, and there may indeed be a temptation to avoid it as an unwelcome addition to the information load imposed by the job. When, however, conditions are rapidly changing, or in the early stages of developing an operation, such feedback will give a flexibility and rapidity of adjustment not otherwise possible.

Taken in conjunction with the limited capacity for decision discussed earlier, considerations of feedback suggest possible reasons for relationships which have been claimed to exist between morale and the size of the working group. It has been argued that a small group is more "democratic," while a large group tends to generate an "authoritarian" leadership which is less acceptable. Evidence about which type of organization leads to better results and greater job satisfaction is, however, conflicting. A possible reconciliation is provided by the results likely to follow if a group generates more information than a single leader can deal with. In the terms we have been using, a "democratic" system means that there is a possibility of effective feedback from group members to leader, whereas an "authoritarian" system means that members of the group are unable to influence the leader's decisions.

As we have seen in Chapters 5 and 7, one reaction to overload in laboratory tasks is that subjects shed part of the load by ignoring some of the signals they should observe and omitting some of the actions they should take. Usually these are the less frequent ones, so that subjects concentrate on the main features of the task and ignore side issues. In this way, they often manage to put up a reasonable, although not, of course, wholly adequate performance.

One way in which an overloaded leader could readily "shed load" would be to rely on routines established in the group to keep it functioning while ignoring feedback from the members. Thus in effect, leadership would become "authoritarian." Its doing so would doubtless have little adverse effect immediately, so that for a while it would seem to be working well, but an important means of recognizing the need for modification or change would have been lost, and the group's performance would therefore tend to become progressively less effective.

Two further applications of feedback theory to social interaction deserve attention as providing an approach to phenomena otherwise difficult to understand.

Behavior of crowds

One of the traditionally difficult problems of social psychology is to account for the uniformity of the behavior of crowds. Obviously crowds produce stimulation likely to raise arousal level which will, in signal-detection theory terms, lower β. This would not, however, of itself produce uniformity of behavior but rather diversity. To account for uniformity in terms such as "social facilitation" is not truly explanatory, since it is essentially ad hoc, and thus little more than descriptive. The present terms, however, provide the simple hypothesis that, when the members of a crowd are all acting alike, the sight and sound of others provide each individual with a kind of augmented feedback of his or her own behavior. This would be especially so if the crowd was, say, shouting slogans in unison. An analogue on a smaller scale is the feeling of "unusual power" reported by crews of rowing eights when their boats are going well; when all are pulling precisely together each man is said to get the feeling that the whole result is due to his own effort. The seeming ratio of effect to effort is thus greatly enhanced, and it is reasonable to suppose that the satisfaction gained from the activity is correspondingly increased.

Friendship, hostility, and loneliness

Perhaps the most far-reaching consequence of feedback in social situations is its role in friendship and hostility, understanding of which in psychological terms has been remarkably elusive (Welford, 1971a). By way of example, let us consider the case of casual friendly acquaintance at a party, where conversation flows between two people with growing mutual approval. Four things seem to be characteristic of this situation. First, each speaker obviously understands what the other is saying, not only in the sense that they talk the same language, but that they code or conceive of objects and events in ways which they both comprehend. Second, the two speakers are roughly matched in the pace at which they produce their ideas, so that neither overloads the other by going too fast, nor bores the other by going too slowly. Third, each is able and willing to adapt remarks to the other, in the sense of modifying statements and behavior in the light of the replies and behavior of the other—in short, each is sensitive to feedback from the other. Fourth, each, in the ideas produced, supplements or complements those of the other. Although they may not always agree, each obtains a set of ideas larger than he or she could produce alone, and is thus able to think more easily, more constructively, or with greater satisfaction. Both thus stimulate each other; in our present terms, the feedback between them is positive. This may not always be so in more mature friendships, where a person may sometimes speak or act to criticize or discourage a friend. In such cases, however, the restraint seems to be a temporary phase within a larger, long-term framework of mutual encouragement and facilitation.

Hostility seems to involve processes which are, broadly speaking, the reverse of those found in friendship. Conversation and other activities, such as fighting between enemies, may produce temporary exchanges in which each reacts to the other and observes the other's reactions, thus securing a feedback situation. Sophisticated forms of hostility may include simulated friendship, with spells in which each leads the other on to greater and greater response. However, the long-term aim of one or both parties in all cases is to reduce the other to a state in which he or she is unable to act or retires from the scene, so that feedback ceases.

While, therefore, friendship is fundamentally constructive and expansive, hostility is essentially destructive. It is true that the rivalry that hostility produces can be stimulating, so that just as scientific advances may come more rapidly in war than in peacetime, individual enemies may spur each other to achievements they would otherwise never have attained. In such cases, however, extra achievement is usually offset to an appreciable extent by the waste of effort and loss of time incurred by one or both parties in trying to undo each other's work, and by losses to third parties who may have been directly or indirectly affected. It can, indeed, be suggested in passing that one of the outstanding problems of human relationships is to secure the stimulating effects of rivalry within an overall framework of friendship: in other words, to compete in achievement without trying at the same time to lower the achievement of others.

If friendship is a relationship of positive feedback and hostility of negative, it seems reasonable to conceive of *loneliness* as a state in which no effective feedback of either kind is present. Thus severe loneliness is often seen in people who have migrated to a country where they do not understand the language well so that easy, lighthearted communication with others is difficult. Less severe loneliness may occur in those who move to a different town or district, away from neighbors and family with whom they have previously had frequent exchanges; even if these were often hostile, they may be recognized as more enlivening than none at all. What can be construed as a further form of loneliness is the alienation between parents and children that seems to go with addiction to television and the consequent breakdown of family conversation. Perhaps the best recognized cases of loneliness, however, are found among old people, and it is here that the conditions and possible means of curing loneliness and of improving human relationships generally could probably be studied most easily. Such a study, while of immediate significance for the care of the elderly, would almost certainly have widespread implications for others suffering from loneliness, as well as for organizational methods and structures.

One of the most striking features of loneliness in old people is the complaint of being lonely even when they have frequent visits from friends, relatives, neighbors, and welfare workers. Loneliness in these cases is not a result of physical isolation. Instead it seems to indicate a breakdown of communication between the old person and those around. One obvious possible source of such breakdown is in failure of hearing, especially for the high tones on which the intelligibility of speech mainly depends. This, coupled with central changes which make for difficulty of coding, integrating, and giving meaning to incoming data quickly (see Welford, 1958, 1964), would result in a restriction at the input end. However, most cases of loneliness do not appear to depend on failures of these kinds, but rather on self-centeredness and restriction of interests which lead to communications from other people being ignored. Communication may be somewhat better with members of the family with whom memories can be shared and subtle nuances understood, and this is probably why old people usually prefer the company of their families to that of outsiders.

The restrictions of input have their counterparts at the output end. For instance, narrow and self-centered interests in the old person will make his or her remarks uninteresting to others. This situation is especially acute in cases of chronic dependence, when demands for attention can make the old person's communications unacceptable. It is perhaps not surprising in such cases that when an old person persistently demands attention without sharing the interests of others, those around are liable to become hostile.

As regards practical action to avoid loneliness and develop social skills, we can see that certain currently popular practices are in line with the model sketched here. For example, group therapy for psychiatric illness and T-Group or sensitivity training in industry, in which people meet in groups to discuss their personal problems and their reactions to each other, appear to depend for their effectiveness upon participants seeing themselves as others see them. Group members are put in a situation in which they have to take note of the effects of what they say and do upon others, and to listen carefully to the remarks of others to a much greater extent than they would normally. They thus learn to pay attention to, and comprehend, communications from others, and to modify their own words and actions so as to convey their meanings and intentions accurately and effectively to others. The early stages of such group discussions tend to produce hostility since many of the comments made are critical and the feedback is thus negative. Later, as participants come to understand each other—and themselves—better, social skills develop and exchanges tend to become more encouraging and thus conducive to friendship.

Social stimulation

Other people are obviously a source of input which is likely to increase arousal. This is partly a direct result of sensory stimulation produced by the mere sight, sound, and touch of others, and partly because their behavior is almost certain to impinge to some extent, demanding some kind of response. Other persons are, in fact, potential sources of the stimulation, uncertainty, and conflict which we noted in the last chapter as raising arousal levels. It is thus understandable that vigilance in a monotonous task is improved by the presence of another person in the same room (e.g., Fraser, 1953), since this tends to offset the lowering of arousal that would otherwise occur. Similarly, the inertness often shown by people living in isolation, such as old people living alone or bedridden in single hospital rooms, may be avoided when several share a home or hospital ward.

Social stimulation can, however, be excessive and lead to overarousal. It is well known that animals kept in crowded conditions tend to develop abnormally large adrenal glands and to be overactive and aggressive. The same seems to be true of human beings who live and work in large cities. Presumably the constant stimulation of other people, the noise they produce, the necessity to weave through crowds and to compete for seats on trains or parking for one's car, raise the chronic level of arousal beyond optimum. Several studies of small human groups imply, however, that sheer numbers are not the only significant factor. The effects of crowding depend rather upon the extent to which people are forced into contact and interdependence upon each other (see Haythorn, 1970; McEwen, 1973). It is reasonable to suppose also that the need to fit one's decisions and actions with those of others is a source of complication and constraint in any situation involving collaboration between two or more people. The value of teamwork and joint action will thus depend on a balance between these constraints, the good or bad effects of stimulation, and the greater achievement that cooperation may bring.

The stimulation derived from interaction with others makes it under-standable that extraversion and introversion are linked with low and high levels of arousal respectively. We have already noted that extraverts tend to seek stimulation. An important source of such stimulation is social, so that turning outwards to make contact with others is an adaptive reaction, tending to raise an unduly low level of arousal to optimum. Introverts, on the other hand, show a similarly adaptive attempt to reduce stimulation by shunning lively social contacts in favor of solitude or a restricted companion-ship.

The needs of individuals seem to be reflected in the norms of societies. An example is seen if one compares Australia and much of the United States and Canada with Europe. In the former, where there are many open spaces and it is relatively easy to be completely alone, it is the norm to visit friends uninvited and to talk to neighbors and to strangers in buses, trains, and restaurants. In Europe, where solitude is more difficult to achieve, such behavior tends to be regarded as an unwarranted invasion of privacy. However, the norm, while it expresses the average need, may cause suffering for some individuals. Thus in Europe, the barriers built up against too much social contact can result in those who do not find social acquaintance easy becoming isolated, while in Australia and North America many introverted people often feel they lack privacy.

The techniques used by individuals to control their social contacts are largely unconscious, but are probably built up and refined by experience and thus deserve to be regarded as skills. Certainly most of us know of techniques we have deliberately used upon occasion to make sure of meeting people we wish to see or of avoiding those we do not. Observations regarding these techniques have until now been made more under the heading of "lifemanship" than of psychology, but the increasing density of population in many countries and cities makes the control of social contact an important and urgent topic for psychological research.

Summary

A close analogy can be drawn between the interaction of an operator with a machine and the social interaction of two or more people. It is thus pertinent to look at social interaction in terms of the chain of processes outlined in Chapter 1.

Social communication depends upon similarity of coding by the parties concerned, not only as regards language but also as regards interests. It further depends on the message being conveyed in ways which enable essential information to be distinguished from irrelevant matter—not always easy in ordinary conversation. Some communications also make excessive demands upon short-term retention. Skills in communication seem to depend upon the perceptual and other coding capacities discussed in previous chapters. Effects of failure to communicate can be seen in some of the problems of race relations, and the present model has suggestions to make in this regard. Codings tend to crystallize into social norms which, once formed, change only slowly, so that any attempt to change them quickly may lead to oscillation.

Capacity for communication depends on the rate at which information can be handled, as discussed in Chapter 4. This has important implications for communications in industry; not only do the chains of communication need to be plotted, but also the loads upon individuals who form the various links. The problem is well illustrated by considerations of leadership in relation to size of group and working conditions: the size of group that can be led by one person is limited by the amount of data the leader can handle from the group members and from the work they are doing. Skill at keeping rate of information within manageable limits can be seen in the selection and coding of input data and output action.

Perhaps the most important factor in the analogy between social interaction and the operation of machines by men is in the role of feedback. Effective feedback is seen to be an essential feature of flexibility in industrial organization and leadership. The uniformity of the behavior of crowds can be understood in terms of the augmented feedback each member obtains from others. Essential differences between friendship and hostility can be defined as positive feedback in the former and negative feedback in the latter. In the same terms, loneliness can be seen as a lack of feedback either positive or negative. Loneliness appears to have little to do with physical isolation, but is rather to be understood in terms of failure to receive communications from others, or to generate communications others are willing to receive.

Techniques such as group therapy and T-Group training can be construed as attempts to increase feedback, and thus to reveal people to themselves as others see them.

Other people are a source of sensory stimulation, uncertainty, and potential or actual conflict, all of which are likely to raise arousal level. Several types of social behavior can be regarded as attempts to prevent arousal level from becoming excessive. Such behaviors appear not only in individuals but in the norms of different communities.

Postscript

The psychologists who, during World War II, left their university laboratories to carry out research on human factors in the operation of military equipment, found the theories they took with them to be of little help as guides to the solution of real-life problems. Looking back, we can see that the reason lay in the way psychology had developed during the preceding decades of the present century. The various branches of the subject—physiological, experimental, social, psychometric, and so on—had all grown independently and in doing so had formulated different principles and terminologies. At the same time, much of what was designated as theory was descriptive rather than explanatory. Between psychology and its neighboring areas of study, cleavages were still deeper. Physiology commanded respect by psychologists, and there were some notable researches done by those who spanned both disciplines, but most physiologists had little interest in psychology. The newly developing subject of sociology was too much involved with the task of establishing its own position to be willing to learn much from psychology, and psychologists found its concepts and terminology lacking in precision.

The "skills approach" which developed from the 1940s on grew essentially from the collaboration of psychologists with engineers who brought mathematical and cybernetic models to the study of human performance. The importance of these models lay in their not being tied to any particular discipline. They apply in principle to the physical sciences as well as to the biological, and within the biological sciences to others as well as psychology. They have thus provided a common framework of ideas and language within which different disciplines find themselves able to communicate more effectively than they have ever been able to do before—a framework which has, moreover, stood up to the acid test of application. Within the different branches of psychology, this style of thinking has profoundly affected physiological and human experimental psychology, and is now beginning to expand and consolidate tentative approaches made in earlier years to areas of social psychology, psychopathology, and psychometrics. In these it still has a long way to go, but it seems fair to claim that what has already been done makes good sense and provides a more precise and quantitative treatment of social and pathological processes than has been available before.

In the wider field of human biology, the skills approach has emphasized the position of psychology as intermediate between the social sciences on the one hand and the older human biological disciplines on the other. In their studies of individual human behavior, psychologists recognize that certain social factors may exert important effects. On the other hand, they know that they are studying a biological organism whose behavior is based on a nervous system reacting to the environment via sense organs and muscles and that they must sooner or later look to physiology for their explanations. Both physiologist and psychologist recognize that these explanations are not at present available and indeed that the goal is not fully attainable because the detailed breakdown of behavior into physiological terms would be impossibly complex. The division between the two disciplines is nevertheless arbitrary and exists essentially in the size of unit studied—for psychology, the whole organism; for physiology, individual cells and structures. In many ways this division is both convenient and necessary; nevertheless, there are occasions when the psychologist must consider the detailed mechanism of the human brain and body in order to tie together many facts which at first sight appear disconnected or even discordant. At the same time, the physiologist considering the action of large masses of nerve cells must often resort to the study of behavior at the level normally within the realm of psychology. Thus there is a two-way traffic between the disciplines in which psychology seeks theory and explanation downwards, and physiology seeks the testing of hypotheses upwards in the scale of functional units.

It is reasonable to suggest that psychology can and should play the same role in relation to social studies as physiology does in relation to psychology, providing the means of conceptualizing the detailed mechanisms of the behavior of groups and organized social units. For psychology to play this role, however, the principle must be recognized that social units are composed of individuals, and that it is their interaction with their environment and each other that produces social phenomena. Such recognition implies that accounts of social phenomena need to be broken down from steady states or slow changes into processes in which, ideally, chains of detailed individual actions can be described. It is often impossible to make this kind of breakdown, just as it is impossible to analyze individual behavior into detailed physiological processes, but the attempt needs to be made and, even if it fails for a time, the ultimate aim must be acknowledged. The psychologist in turn must remember that, just as psychological findings have sometimes pointed to matters requiring physiological research, so social studies are likely to direct the psychologist's attention to problems in his own field that might otherwise pass unnoticed.

The way seems open for a unification of the human biological and social sciences on a much wider basis than has existed before. The greatest barrier to such unification in the past appears to have been the vast array of concepts, principles, and terms that would have to be mastered by anyone attempting to bring them together. We can, perhaps, hope that the provision of a relatively small set of concepts and terms which span the whole range can be regarded not as just one more terminology to be mastered but as providing the simplification that will make the wider mastery possible.

Appendix

Table A 1. *Normal deviates and ordinates for calculating d' and β when the varianc of the distributions being compared are equal*

p	Normal deviate	Ordinate	p	Normal deviate	Ordinate
0.0	0.0	0.0	.21	.806	.288
.001	3.090	.003	.22	.772	.296
.002	2.878	.006	.23	.739	.304
.003	2.748	.009	.24	.706	.311
.004	2.652	.012	.25	.674	.318
.005	2.576	.015	.26	.643	.325
.006	2.512	.017	.27	.613	.331
.007	2.457	.020	.28	.583	.337
.008	2.409	.022	.29	.553	.342
.009	2.366	.024	.30	.524	.348
.01	2.326	.027	.31	.496	.353
.02	2.054	.048	.32	.468	.358
.03	1.881	.068	.33	.440	.362
.04	1.751	.086	.34	.412	.367
.05	1.645	.103	.35	.385	.371
.06	1.555	.119	.36	.358	.374
.07	1.476	.134	.37	.332	.378
.08	1.405	.149	.38	.305	.381
.09	1.341	.162	.39	.279	.384
.10	1.282	.176	.40	.253	.386
.11	1.227	.188	.41	.228	.389
.12	1.175	.200	.42	.202	.391
.13	1.126	.212	.43	.176	.393
.14	1.080	.223	.44	.151	.394
.15	1.036	.233	.45	.126	.396
.16	.994	.243	.46	.100	.397
.17	.954	.253	.47	.075	.398
.18	.915	.263	.48	.050	.398
.19	.878	.272	.49	.025	.399
.20	.842	.280	.50	.000	.399

To obtain d', add the normal deviates corresponding to the proportions (p) of misses and false positives, i.e.,

$$d' = ND \text{ for } pNO_{SN} + ND \text{ for } pYES_N$$

To obtain β, divide the ordinate corresponding to the proportion (p) of misses by the ordinate corresponding to the proportion (p) of false positives, i.e.,

$$\beta = \frac{\text{Ordinate for } pNO_{SN}}{\text{Ordinate for } pYES_N}$$

Table A 2. *Log₂ n for numbers from 1 to 100*

n	$\log_2 n$	n	$\log_2 n$	n	$\log_2 n$	n	$\log_2 n$
1	0.000	26	4.700	51	5.672	76	6.248
2	1.000	27	4.755	52	5.700	77	6.267
3	1.585	28	4.807	53	5.728	78	6.285
4	2.000	29	4.858	54	5.755	79	6.304
5	2.322	30	4.907	55	5.781	80	6.322
6	2.585	31	4.954	56	5.807	81	6.340
7	2.807	32	5.000	57	5.833	82	6.358
8	3.000	33	5.044	58	5.858	83	6.375
9	3.170	34	5.087	59	5.883	84	6.392
10	3.322	35	5.129	60	5.907	85	6.409
11	3.459	36	5.170	61	5.931	86	6.426
12	3.585	37	5.209	62	5.954	87	6.443
13	3.700	38	5.248	63	5.977	88	6.459
14	3.807	39	5.285	64	6.000	89	6.476
15	3.907	40	5.322	65	6.022	90	6.492
16	4.000	41	5.358	66	6.044	91	6.508
17	4.087	42	5.392	67	6.066	92	6.524
18	4.170	43	5.426	68	6.087	93	6.539
19	4.248	44	5.459	69	6.109	94	6.555
20	4.322	45	5.492	70	6.129	95	6.570
21	4.392	46	5.523	71	6.150	96	6.585
22	4.459	47	5.555	72	6.170	97	6.600
23	4.524	48	5.585	73	6.190	98	6.615
24	4.585	49	5.615	74	6.209	99	6.629
25	4.644	50	5.644	75	6.229	100	6.644

Table A 3. $p \log_2 \left(\dfrac{1}{p} \right)$

p	$p \log_2 \left(\dfrac{1}{p} \right)$	p	$p \log_2 \left(\dfrac{1}{p} \right)$
.01	.066	.51	.495
.02	.113	.52	.491
.03	.152	.53	.485
.04	.186	.54	.480
.05	.216	.55	.474
.06	.244	.56	.468
.07	.269	.57	.462
.08	.292	.58	.456
.09	.313	.59	.449
.10	.332	.60	.442
.11	.350	.61	.435
.12	.367	.62	.427
.13	.383	.63	.420
.14	.397	.64	.412
.15	.411	.65	.404
.16	.423	.66	.396
.17	.435	.67	.387
.18	.445	.68	.378
.19	.455	.69	.369
.20	.464	.70	.360
.21	.473	.71	.351
.22	.481	.72	.341
.23	.488	.73	.331
.24	.494	.74	.321
.25	.500	.75	.311
.26	.505	.76	.301
.27	.510	.77	.290
.28	.514	.78	.280
.29	.518	.79	.269
.30	.521	.80	.258
.31	.524	.81	.246
.32	.526	.82	.235
.33	.528	.83	.223
.34	.529	.84	.211
.35	.530	.85	.199
.36	.531	.86	.187
.37	.531	.87	.175
.38	.530	.88	.162
.39	.530	.89	.150
.40	.529	.90	.137
.41	.527	.91	.124
.42	.526	.92	.111
.43	.524	.93	.097
.44	.521	.94	.084
.45	.518	.95	.070
.46	.515	.96	.057
.47	.512	.97	.043
.48	.508	.98	.029
.49	.504	.99	.014
.50	.500	1.00	0.0

Table A 4. $p \log_2 \left(\dfrac{1}{p} \right)$ for certain sets of fractions not obtainable from Table A 3.

Fraction	$p \log_2 \left(\dfrac{1}{p} \right)$	Fraction	$p \log_2 \left(\dfrac{1}{p} \right)$
1/3	.528	1/11	.314
2/3	.390	2/11	.447
		3/11	.511
1/6	.431	4/11	.531
2/6	.528	5/11	.517
3/6	.500	6/11	.477
4/6	.390	7/11	.415
5/6	.219	8/11	.334
		9/11	.237
1/7	.401	10/11	.136
2/7	.516		
3/7	.524	1/12	.298
4/7	.462	2/12	.431
5/7	.347	3/12	.500
6/7	.191	4/12	.528
		5/12	.526
1/8	.375	6/12	.500
2/8	.500	7/12	.454
3/8	.531	8/12	.390
4/8	.500	9/12	.311
5/8	.424	10/12	.219
6/8	.311	11/12	.115
7/8	.169		
		1/13	.284
1/9	.352	2/13	.415
2/9	.482	3/13	.488
3/9	.528	4/13	.523
4/9	.520	5/13	.530
5/9	.471	6/13	.515
6/9	.390	7/13	.481
7/9	.282	8/13	.431
8/9	.151	9/13	.367
		10/13	.291
		11/13	.204
		12/13	.106

References

Abbey, D. S. Control-display-subject interaction and performance on a complex perceptual-motor task. *Ergonomics*, 1964, *7*, 151-164.

Adams, J. A. Multiple versus single problem training in human problem solving. *Journal of Experimental Psychology*, 1954, *48*, 15-18.

Adams, J. A. A source of decrement in psychomotor performance. *Journal of Experimental Psychology*, 1955, *49*, 390-394.

Adams, J. A. A closed-loop theory of motor learning. *Journal of Motor Behavior*, 1971, *3*, 111-150.

Adams, J. A., & Bray, N. W. A closed-loop theory of paired-associate verbal learning. *Psychological Review*, 1970, *77*, 385-405.

Adams, J. A., & Dijkstra, S. Short-term memory for motor responses. *Journal of Experimental Psychology*, 1966, *71*, 314-318.

Adams, J. A., & Goetz, E. T. Feedback and practice as variables in error detection and correction. *Journal of Motor Behavior*, 1973, *5*, 217-224.

Adams, J. A., Goetz, E. T., & Marshall, P. H. Response feedback and motor learning. *Journal of Experimental Psychology*, 1972, *92*, 391-397.

Alegria, J., & Bertelson, P. Time uncertainty, number of alternatives and particular signal-response pair as determinants of choice reaction time. *Acta Psychologica*, 1970, *33*, 36-44.

Anderson, N. H. Averaging of space and number stimuli with simultaneous presentation. *Journal of Experimental Psychology*, 1968, *77*, 383-392.

Andjus, R. K., Knopfelmacher, F., Russell, R. W., & Smith, A. U. Some effects of severe hypothermia on learning and retention. *Quarterly Journal of Experimental Psychology*, 1956, *8*, 15-23.

Annett, J. Learning a pressure under conditions of immediate and delayed knowledge of results. *Quarterly Journal of Experimental Psychology*, 1959, *11*, 3-15.

Annett, J. The role of action feedback in the acquisition of simple motor responses. *Journal of Motor Behavior*, 1970, *2*, 217-221.

Annett, J., Golby, C. W., & Kay, H. The measurement of elements in an assembly task—the information output of the human motor system. *Quarterly Journal of Experimental Psychology*, 1958, *10*, 1-11.

Annett, J., & Kay, H. Knowledge of results and "skilled performance." *Occupational Psychology*, 1957, *31*, 69-79.

Archer, E. J., Kent, G. W., & Mote, F. A. Effect of long-term practice and time-on-target information feedback on a complex tracking task. *Journal of Experimental Psychology*, 1956, *51*, 103-112.

Archer, E. J., & Namikas, G. A. Pursuit rotor performance as a function of delay of information feedback. *Journal of Experimental Psychology*, 1958, *56*, 325-327.

Argyle, M. *The Psychology of Interpersonal Behaviour*. Harmondsworth: Penguin, 1967.

Attneave, F. Some informational aspects of visual perception. *Psychological Review*, 1954, *61*, 183-193.

Attneave, F. Transfer of experience with a class-schema to identification-learning of patterns and shapes. *Journal of Experimental Psychology*, 1957, *54*, 81–88.

.bach, E., & Sperling, G. Short-term storage of information in vision. In C. Cherry (Ed.), *Information Theory: Fourth London Symposium*. London: Butterworth, 1961. (Pp. 196–211.)

Bachem, A. Note on Neu's review of the literature on absolute pitch. *Psychological Bulletin*, 1948, *45*, 161–162.

Baddeley, A. D. Language-habits, S-R compatibility, and verbal learning. *American Journal of Psychology*, 1964, *77*, 463–468.

Baddeley, A. D. The influence of acoustic and semantic similarity on long-term memory for word sequences. *Quarterly Journal of Experimental Psychology*, 1966a, *18*, 302–309.

Baddeley, A. D. Short-term memory for word sequences as a function of acoustic, semantic and formal similarity. *Quarterly Journal of Experimental Psychology*, 1966b, *18*, 362–365.

Baddeley, A. D., & Ecob, J. R. Reaction time and short-term memory: Implications of repetition effects for the high-speed exhaustive scan hypothesis. *Quarterly Journal of Experimental Psychology*, 1973, *25*, 229–240.

Baker, C. H., & Young, P. Feedback during training and retention of motor skills. *Canadian Journal of Psychology*, 1960, *14*, 257–264.

Bartlett, F. C. *Remembering*. London: Cambridge University Press, 1932.

Bartlett, F. C. Fatigue following highly skilled work. *Proceedings of the Royal Society*, B, 1943, *131*, 247–257.

Bartlett, F. C. The measurement of human skill. *British Medical Journal*, 1947, i, 835 & 877. Reprinted *Occupational Psychology*, 1948, *22*, 31–38 and 83–91.

Bartley, S. H., & Chute, E. *Fatigue and Impairment in Man*. New York & London: McGraw-Hill, 1947.

Batten, D. E. Recall of paired associates as a function of arousal and recall interval. *Perceptual and Motor Skills*, 1967, *24*, 1055–1058.

Beishon, R. J. Problems of task description in process control. *Ergonomics*, 1967, *10*, 177–186.

Bekesy, G. von. *Sensory Inhibition*. Princeton: Princeton University Press, 1967.

Belbin, E. The influence of interpolated recall upon recognition. *Quarterly Journal of Experimental Psychology*, 1950, *2*, 163–169.

Belbin, E. Methods of training older workers. *Ergonomics*, 1958, *1*, 207–221.

Belbin, E. *Training the Adult Worker*. D.S.I.R. Problems of Progress in Industry No. 15. London: H.M.S.O., 1964.

Belbin, E., Belbin, R. M., & Hill, F. A comparison between the results of three different methods of operator training. *Ergonomics*, 1957, *1*, 39–50.

Belbin, E., & Downs, S. M. Activity learning and the older worker. *Ergonomics*, 1964, *7*, 429–437.

Belbin, E., & Downs, S. Teaching paired associates: The problem of age. *Occupational Psychology*, 1966, *40*, 67–74.

Belbin, R. M. *The Discovery Method: An International Experiment in Retraining*. Paris: O.E.C.D., 1969.

Berger, C., & Mahneke, A. Fatigue in two simple visual tasks. *American Journal of Psychology*, 1954, *67*, 509–512.

Berlyne, D. E., Borsa, D. M., Hamacher, J. H., & Koenig, I. D. V. Paired-associate learning and the timing of arousal. *Journal of Experimental Psychology*, 1966, *72*, 1–6.

Bertelson, P. Sequential redundancy and speed in a serial two-choice responding task. *Quarterly Journal of Experimental Psychology*, 1961, *13*, 90–102.

Bertelson, P. S-R relationships and reaction times to new versus repeated signals in a serial task. *Journal of Experimental Psychology*, 1963, *65*, 478–484.

Bertelson, P. Serial choice reaction-time as a function of response versus signal-and-response repetition. *Nature*, 1965, *206*, 217–218.

Bertelson, P. Central intermittency twenty years later. *Quarterly Journal of Experimental Psychology*, 1966, *18*, 153–163.

Bertelson, P., & Joffe, R. Blockings in prolonged serial responding. *Ergonomics*, 1963, *6*, 109–116.

Bertelson, P., & Renkin, A. Reaction times to new versus repeated signals in a serial task as a function of response-signal time interval. *Acta Psychologica*, 1966, *25*, 132–136.

Besrest, A., & Requin, J. Development of expectancy wave and time course of preparatory set in a simple reaction-time task: Preliminary results. In S. Kornblum (Ed.), *Attention and Performance IV*. New York: Academic Press, 1973. (Pp. 209–219.)

Bills, A. G. The influence of muscular tension on the efficiency of mental work. *American Journal of Psychology*, 1927, *38*, 227–251.

Bills, A. G. Blocking: A new principle in mental fatigue. *American Journal of Psychology*, 1931, *43*, 230–245.

Bilodeau, E. A., & Bilodeau, I. McD. (Eds.). *Principles of Skill Acquisition*. New York: Academic Press, 1969.

Bilodeau, E. A., Jones, M. B., & Levy, C. M. Long-term memory as a function of retention time and repeated recalling. *Journal of Experimental Psychology*, 1964, *67*, 303–309.

Bilodeau, I. McD., & Rosenquist, H. S. Supplementary feedback in rotary-pursuit tracking. *Journal of Experimental Psychology*, 1964, *68*, 53–57.

Binet, A., & Henri, V. La mémoire des mots. *Année Psychologique*, 1894, *1*, 1–23.

Blake, M. J. F. Relationship between circadian rhythm of body temperature and introversion-extraversion. *Nature*, 1967, *215*, 896–897.

Blyth, K. W. Ipsilateral confusion in 2-choice and 4-choice responses with the hands and feet. *Nature*, 1963, *199*, 1312.

Blyth, K. W. Errors in a further four-choice reaction task with the hands and feet. *Nature*, 1964, *201*, 641–642.

Boswell, J. J., & Bilodeau, E. A. Short-term retention of a simple motor task as a function of interpolated activity. *Perceptual and Motor Skills*, 1964, *18*, 227–230.

Bradley, J. V. Direction-of-knob-turn stereotypes. *Journal of Applied Psychology*, 1959, *43*, 21–24.

Brainard, R. W., Irby, T. S., Fitts, P. M., & Alluisi, E. A. Some variables influencing the rate of gain of information. *Journal of Experimental Psychology*, 1962, *63*, 105–110.

Brebner, J. S-R compatibility and changes in RT with practice. *Acta Psychologica*, 1973, *37*, 93–106.

Brebner, J., & Gordon, I. Ensemble size and selective response times with a constant signal rate. *Quarterly Journal of Experimental Psychology*, 1962, *14*, 113–116.

Brebner, J., & Gordon, I. The influence of signal probability and the number of non-signal categories on selective response times. *Quarterly Journal of Experimental Psychology*, 1964, *16*, 56–60.

Brebner, J., Shephard, M., & Cairney, P. Spatial relationships and S-R compatibility. *Acta Psychologica*, 1972, *36*, 1-15.

Bricker, P. D. The identification of redundant stimulus patterns. *Journal of Experimental Psychology*, 1955, *49*, 73-81.

Briggs, G. E. On the predictor variable for choice reaction time. *Memory and Cognition*, 1974, *2*, 575-580.

Briggs, G. E., & Swanson, J. M. Encoding, decoding, and central functions in human information processing. *Journal of Experimental Psychology*, 1970, *86*, 296-308.

Briggs, G. E., & Waters, L. K. Training and transfer as a function of component interaction. *Journal of Experimental Psychology*, 1958, *56*, 492-500.

Broadbent, D. E. Speaking and listening simultaneously. *Journal of Experimental Psychology*, 1952, *43*, 267-273.

Broadbent, D. E. The role of auditory localization in attention and memory span. *Journal of Experimental Psychology*, 1954, *47*, 191-196.

Broadbent, D. E. Immediate memory and simultaneous stimuli. *Quarterly Journal of Experimental Psychology*, 1957, *9*, 1-11.

Broadbent, D. E. *Perception and Communication*. London: Pergamon Press, 1958.

Broadbent, D. E. *Decision and Stress*. London: Academic Press, 1971.

Broadbent, D. E., & Gregory, M. Vigilance considered as a statistical decision. *British Journal of Psychology*, 1963, *54*, 309-323.

Brown, C. H. The relation of magnitude of galvanic skin responses and resistance levels to the rate of learning. *Journal of Experimental Psychology*, 1937, *20*, 262-278.

Brown, I. D. Measuring the ''spare mental capacity'' of car drivers by a subsidiary auditory task. *Ergonomics*, 1962, *5*, 247-250.

Brown, I. D. A comparison of two subsidiary tasks used to measure fatigue in car drivers. *Ergonomics*, 1965a, *8*, 467-473.

Brown, I. D. Effect of a car radio on driving in traffic. *Ergonomics*, 1965b, *8*, 475-479.

Brown, I. D., & Poulton, E. C. Measuring the spare ''mental capacity'' of car drivers by a subsidiary task. *Ergonomics*, 1961, *4*, 35-40.

Brown, I. D., Tickner, A. H., & Simmonds, D. C. V. Interference between concurrent tasks of driving and telephoning. *Journal of Applied Psychology*, 1969, *53*, 419-424.

Brown, J. Some tests of the decay theory of immediate memory. *Quarterly Journal of Experimental Psychology*, 1958, *10*, 12-21.

Bruce, R. W. Conditions of transfer of training. *Journal of Experimental Psychology*, 1933, *16*, 343-361.

Bryan, W. L., & Harter, N. Studies in the physiology and psychology of the telegraphic language. *Psychological Review*, 1897, *4*, 27-53.

Bryan, W. L., & Harter, N. Studies on the telegraphic language. The acquisition of a hierarchy of habits. *Psychological Review*, 1899, *6*, 345-375.

Bursill, A. E. The restriction of peripheral vision during exposure to hot and humid conditions. *Quarterly Journal of Experimental Psychology*, 1958, *10*, 113-129.

Callantine, M. F., & Warren, J. M. Learning sets in human concept formation. *Psychological Reports*, 1955, *1*, 363-367.

Carmichael, L., Hogan, H. P., & Walter, A. A. An experimental study of the effect of language on the reproduction of visually perceived form. *Journal of Experimental Psychology*, 1932, *15*, 73-86.

Carpenter, A. A case of absolute pitch. *Quarterly Journal of Experimental Psychology*, 1951, *3*, 92-93.

Cattell, J. M. On errors of observation. *American Journal of Psychology*, 1893, *5*, 285-293.

Chown, S., Belbin, E., & Downs, S. Programmed instruction as a method of teaching paired associates to older learners. *Journal of Gerontology*, 1967, *22*, 212-219.

Christie, L. S., & Luce, R. D. Decision structure and time relations in simple choice behaviour. *Bulletin of Mathematical Biophysics*, 1956, *18*, 89-111.

Clay, H. M. *Research in Relation to Operator Training*. Monograph available from the Librarian, Science Research Council, London W.C.1, 1964.

Colquhoun, W. P. Temperament, inspection efficiency, and time of day. *Ergonomics*, 1960, *3*, 377-378.

Colquhoun, W. P., & Corcoran, D. W. J. The effects of time of day and social isolation on the relationship between temperament and performance. *British Journal of Social and Clinical Psychology*, 1964, *3*, 226-231.

Conrad, R. Speed and load stress in sensorimotor skill. *British Journal of Industrial Medicine*, 1951, *8*, 1-7.

Conrad, R. Missed signals in a sensorimotor skill. *Journal of Experimental Psychology*, 1954a, *48*, 1-9.

Conrad, R. Speed stress. In W. F. Floyd & A. T. Welford (Eds.), *Symposium on Human Factors in Equipment Design*. London: H. K. Lewis & Co. for the Ergonomics Research Society, 1954b. (Pp. 95-102.)

Conrad, R. Practice, familiarity, and reading rate for words and nonsense syllables. *Quarterly Journal of Experimental Psychology*, 1962, *14*, 71-76.

Corcoran, D. W. J. An acoustic factor in letter cancellation. *Nature*, 1966, *210*, 658.

Corcoran, D. W. J. Acoustic factor in proofreading. *Nature*, 1967a, *214*, 851-852.

Corcoran, D. W. J. Serial and parallel classification. *British Journal of Psychology*, 1967b, *58*, 197-203.

Corcoran, D. W. J., & Weening, D. L. Acoustic factors in visual search. *Quarterly Journal of Experimental Psychology*, 1968, *20*, 83-85.

Corkin, S. Acquisition of motor skill after bilateral medial temporal-lobe excision. *Neuropsychologia*, 1968, *6*, 255-265.

Courts, F. A. Relations between experimentally induced muscular tension and memorization. *Journal of Experimental Psychology*, 1939, *25*, 235-256.

Crafts, L. W., & Gilbert, R. W. The effect of knowledge of results on maze learning and retention. *Journal of Educational Psychology*, 1935, *26*, 177-187.

Craik, K. J. W. Theory of the human operator in control systems II. Man as an element in a control system. *British Journal of Psychology*, 1948, *38*, 142-148.

Crawford, A. Fatigue and driving. *Ergonomics*, 1961, *4*, 143-154.

Crossman, E. R. F. W. Entropy and choice time: The effect of frequency unbalance on choice-response. *Quarterly Journal of Experimental Psychology*, 1953, *5*, 41-51.

Crossman, E. R. F. W. The information capacity of the human operator in symbolic and nonsymbolic control processes. In *Information Theory and the Human Operator*. Ministry of Supply Publication WR/D2/56, 1956.

Crossman, E. R. F. W. A theory of the acquisition of speed-skill. *Ergonomics*, 1959, *2*, 153-166.

Crossman, E. R. F. W. *Automation and Skill*. D.S.I.R. Problems of Progress in Industry No. 9. London: H.M.S.O., 1960.

Crossman, E. R. F. W. Information and serial order in human immediate memory. In C. Cherry (Ed.), *Information Theory*. London: Butterworth & Co., 1961. (Pp. 147-159.)

Crossman, E. R. F. W., & Goodeve, P. J. Feedback control of hand-movement and Fitts' law. Communication to the Experimental Psychology Society, 1963.

Dale, H. C. A. Retroactive interference in short-term memory. *Nature*, 1964, *203*, 1408.

Dale, H. C. A. Familiarity and free recall. *Quarterly Journal of Experimental Psychology*, 1967, *19*, 103-108.

Dardano, J. F. Relationships of intermittent noise, intersignal interval, and skin conductance to vigilance behavior. *Journal of Applied Psychology*, 1962, *46*, 106-114.

Darrow, C. W. Emotion as relative functional decortication: The role of conflict. *Psychological Review*, 1935, *42*, 566-578.

Davies, D. R., & Tune, G. S. *Human Vigilance Performance*. London: Staples Press, 1970.

Davis, D. R. *Pilot Error*. Air Ministry Publication A.P. 3139A. London: H.M.S.O., 1948.

Davis, D. R. Human errors and transport accidents. *Ergonomics*, 1958, *2*, 24-33.

Davis, D. R. Railway signals passed at danger: The drivers, circumstances and psychological processes. *Ergonomics*, 1966, *9*, 211-222.

Davis, D. R., & Sinha, D. The effect of one experience upon the recall of another. *Quarterly Journal of Experimental Psychology*, 1950, *2*, 43-52.

Davis, R., Moray, N., & Treisman, A. Imitative responses and the rate of gain of information. *Quarterly Journal of Experimental Psychology*, 1961a, *13*, 78-89.

Davis, R., Sutherland, N. S., & Judd, B. R. Information content in recognition and recall. *Journal of Experimental Psychology*, 1961b, *61*, 422-429.

Davis, S. W. Auditory and visual flicker-fusion as measures of fatigue. *American Journal of Psychology*, 1955, *68*, 654-657.

Dees, V., & Grindley, G. C. The effect of knowledge of results on learning and performance IV. The direction of the error in very simple skills. *Quarterly Journal of Experimental Psychology*, 1951, *3*, 36-42.

Delin, P. S. The effect of high and low meaningfulness and interitem association upon the level of difficulty of a serial task. *Psychonomic Science*, 1968a, *12*, 71-72.

Delin, P. S. Success in recall as a function of success in implementation of mnemonic instructions. *Psychonomic Science*, 1968b, *12*, 153-154.

Delin, P. S. The learning to criterion of a serial list with and without mnemonic instructions. *Psychonomic Science*, 1969a, *16*, 169-170.

Delin, P. S. Learning and retention of English words with successive approximations to a complex mnemonic instruction. *Psychonomic Science*, 1969b, *17*, 87-89.

Delin, P. S. The effects of mnemonic instruction and list length on serial learning and retention. *Psychonomic Science*, 1969c, *17*, 111-113.

Delin, P. S. An experiment examining list-learning with and without the mnemonic use of bizarre associations. *Journal of General Psychology*, 1969d, *81*, 249-260.

Dember, W. N., & Earl, R. W. Analysis of exploratory, manipulatory, and curiosity behaviors. *Psychological Review*, 1957, *64*, 91-96.

Donders, F. C. Over de snelheid van psychische processen. *Onderzoekingen gedaan in het Physiologisch Laboratorium der Utrechtsche Hoogeschool*, 1868-1869, *Tweede reeks*, 1868, II, 92-120. Translated by W. G. Koster, On the speed of mental processes. *Acta Psychologica*, 1969, *30*, 412-431.

Duncan, C. P. Transfer after training with single versus multiple tasks. *Journal of*

Experimental Psychology, 1958, *55*, 63–72.

Eagle, M. N. The effect of learning strategies upon free recall. *American Journal of Psychology*, 1967, *80*, 421–425.

Earhard, B. Perception and retention of familiar and unfamiliar material. *Journal of Experimental Psychology*, 1968, *76*, 585–595.

Eason, R. G., Beardshall, A., & Jaffee, S. Performance and physiological indicants of activation in a vigilance situation. *Perceptual and Motor Skills*, 1965, *20*, 3–13.

Eccles, J. C. *The Neurophysiological Basis of Mind*. London: Oxford University Press, 1953.

Edwards, W. Behavioural decision theory. *Annual Review of Psychology*, 1961, *12*, 473–498.

Egeth, H. Selective attention. *Psychological Bulletin*, 1967, *67*, 41–57.

El-Temamy, M. A. A. Unpublished Thesis, University of Birmingham, 1966.

Erdmann, R. L., & Neal, A. S. Word legibility as a function of letter legibility, with word size, word familiarity, and resolution as parameters. *Journal of Applied Psychology*, 1968, *52*, 403–409.

Eriksen, C. W., & Collins, J. F. Sensory traces versus the psychological moment in the temporal organization of form. *Journal of Experimental Psychology*, 1968, *77*, 376–382.

Eysenck, H. J. *The Structure of Human Personality*. London: Methuen, 1965.

Eysenck, H. J. *The Biological Basis of Personality*. Springfield, Illinois: Charles C Thomas, 1970.

Filbey, R. A., & Gazzaniga, M. S. Splitting the normal brain with reaction time. *Psychonomic Science*, 1969, *17*, 335–336.

Fine, B. J. Introversion-extraversion and motor vehicle driver behavior. *Perceptual and Motor Skills*, 1963, *12*, 95–100.

Fitts, P. M. The information capacity of the human motor system in controlling the amplitude of movement. *Journal of Experimental Psychology*, 1954, *47*, 381–391.

Fitts, P. M. Cognitive aspects of information processing: III. Set for speed versus accuracy. *Journal of Experimental Psychology*, 1966, *71*, 849–857.

Fitts, P. M., & Seeger, C. M. S-R compatibility: Spatial characteristics of stimulus and response codes. *Journal of Experimental Psychology*, 1953, *46*, 199–210.

Fitts, P. M., & Switzer, G. Cognitive aspects of information processing: I. The familiarity of S-R sets and subsets. *Journal of Experimental Psychology*, 1962, *63*, 321–329.

Foster, H. The operation of set in a visual search task. *Journal of Experimental Psychology*, 1962, *63*, 74–83.

Fraser, D. C. The relation of an environmental variable to performance in a prolonged visual task. *Quarterly Journal of Experimental Psychology*, 1953, *5*, 31–32.

Freeman, G. L. The facilitative and inhibitory effects of muscular tension upon performance. *American Journal of Psychology*, 1933, *45*, 17–52.

Freeman, G. L. The relationship between performance level and bodily activity level. *Journal of Experimental Psychology*, 1940, *26*, 602–608.

Freud, S. *The Psychopathology of Everyday Life*. London: Fisher Unwin, 1914.

Furneaux, W. D. The psychologist and the university. *University Quarterly*, 1962, *17*, 33–47.

Garner, W. R., & Gottwald, R. L. The perception and learning of temporal patterns. *Quarterly Journal of Experimental Psychology*, 1968, *20*, 97–109.

Gates, A. I. Recitation as a factor in memorizing. *Archives of Psychology, N.Y.,* 1917, *6,* No. 40.

Gerhard, D. J. The judgement of velocity and prediction of motion. *Ergonomics,* 1959, *2,* 287–304.

Gibbs, C. B. The continuous regulation of skilled response by kinaesthetic feed back. *British Journal of Psychology,* 1954, *45,* 24–39.

Gibbs, C. B. Probability learning in step-input tracking. *British Journal of Psychology,* 1965, *56,* 233–242.

Gibbs, C. B., & Brown, I. D. Increased production from information incentives in an uninteresting repetitive task. *Manager,* 1956, *24,* 374–379.

Gibson, J. J. *The Perception of the Visual World.* Boston, Mass.: Houghton Mifflin, 1950.

Gibson, J. J. What gives rise to the perception of motion? *Psychological Review,* 1968, *75,* 335–346.

Gilinsky, A. S. Perceived size and distance in visual space. *Psychological Review,* 1951, *58,* 460–482.

Glanzer, M., Taub, T., & Murphy, R. An evaluation of three theories of figural organization. *American Journal of Psychology,* 1968, *81,* 53–66.

Glickman, S. E. Perseverative neural processes and consolidation of the memory trace. *Psychological Bulletin,* 1961, *58,* 218–233.

Goldman-Eisler, F. The determinants of the rate of speech output and their mutual relations. *Journal of Psychosomatic Research,* 1956, *2,* 137–143.

Goldman-Eisler, F. Speech production and the predictability of words in context. *Quarterly Journal of Experimental Psychology,* 1958, *10,* 96–106.

Goldman-Eisler, F. Hesitation and information in speech. In C. Cherry (Ed.), *Information Theory.* London: Butterworth, 1961. (Pp. 162–174.)

Goldstein, M., & Rittenhouse, C. H. Knowledge of results in the acquisition and transfer of a gunnery skill. *Journal of Experimental Psychology,* 1954, *48,* 187–196.

Gordon, I. E. Interactions between items in visual search. *Journal of Experimental Psychology,* 1968, *76,* 348–355.

Grandjean, E., & Perret, E. Effects of pupil aperture and of the time of exposure on the fatigue induced variations of the flicker fusion frequency. *Ergonomics,* 1961, *4,* 17–23.

Gray, J. A., & Wedderburn, A. A. I. Grouping strategies with simultaneous stimuli. *Quarterly Journal of Experimental Psychology,* 1960, *12,* 180–184.

Green, D. M., & Swets, J. A. *Signal Detection Theory and Psychophysics.* New York: John Wiley & Sons, 1966.

Gregory, R. L. *Eye and Brain: The Psychology of Seeing.* London: World University Library, 1966.

Griew, S. Information gain in tasks involving different stimulus-response relationships. *Nature,* 1958, *182,* 1819.

Hale, D. J. Sequential effects in a two-choice serial reaction task. *Quarterly Journal of Experimental Psychology,* 1967, *19,* 133–141.

Hamilton, P., & Copeman, A. The effect of alcohol and noise on components of a tracking and monitoring task. *British Journal of Psychology,* 1970, *61,* 149–156.

Harcourt, R. A. F. Personal communication, 1959.

Haythorn, W. W. Interpersonal stress in isolated groups. In J. E. McGrath (Ed.), *Social and Psychological Factors in Stress.* New York: Holt, Rinehart & Winston, 1970. (Pp. 159–176.)

Hebb, D. O. *The Organization of Behavior.* New York: John Wiley & Sons; London: Chapman & Hall, 1949.

Hebb, D. O. Drives and the C.N.S. (Conceptual Nervous System). *Psychological Review,* 1955, *62,* 243-254.

Hebron, M. E. *Motivated Learning: A Developmental Study from Birth to the Senium.* London: Methuen, 1966.

Henderson, A., Goldman-Eisler, F., & Skarbek, A. The common value of pausing time in spontaneous speech. *Quarterly Journal of Experimental Psychology,* 1965, *17,* 343-345.

Herman, L. M., & Kantowitz, B. H. The psychological refractory period effect: Only half the double-stimulation story? *Psychological Bulletin,* 1970, *73,* 74-88.

Hick, W. E. On the rate of gain of information. *Quarterly Journal of Experimental Psychology,* 1952a, *4,* 11-26.

Hick, W. E. Why the human operator? *Transactions of the Society for Instrument Technology,* 1952b, *4,* 67-77.

Hilgendorf, L. Information input and response time. *Ergonomics,* 1966, *9,* 31-37.

Hochberg, J., & McAlister, E. A quantitative approach to figural "goodness." *Journal of Experimental Psychology,* 1953, *46,* 361-364.

Hockey, G. R. J. Effect of loud noise on attentional selectivity. *Quarterly Journal of Experimental Psychology,* 1970a, *22,* 28-36.

Hockey, G. R. J. Signal probability and spatial location as possible bases for increased selectivity in noise. *Quarterly Journal of Experimental Psychology,* 1970b, *22,* 37-42.

Hodge, M. H., & Pollack, I. Confusion matrix analysis of single and multidimensional auditory displays. *Journal of Experimental Psychology,* 1962, *63,* 129-142.

Holding, D. H. Transfer between difficult and easy tasks. *British Journal of Psychology,* 1962, *53,* 397-407.

Holding, D. H., & Macrae, A. W. Guidance, restriction, and knowledge of results. *Ergonomics,* 1964, *7,* 289-295.

Holding, D. H., & Macrae, A. W. Rate and force of guidance in perceptual-motor tasks with reversed or random spatial correspondence. *Ergonomics,* 1966, *9,* 289-296.

Howard, T. C. The relation between psychological and mathematical probability. *American Journal of Psychology,* 1963, *76,* 335.

Howell, W. C., & Kreidler, D. L. Information processing under contradictory instructional sets. *Journal of Experimental Psychology,* 1963, *65,* 39-46.

Hubel, D. H., & Wiesel, T. N. Receptive fields, binocular interaction, and functional architecture in the cat's visual cortex. *Journal of Physiology,* 1962, *160,* 106-154.

Hubel, D. H., & Wiesel, T. N. Receptive fields and functional architecture of monkey striate cortex. *Journal of Physiology,* 1968, *195,* 215-243.

Hulbert, S. F. Drivers' GSRs in traffic. *Perceptual and Motor Skills,* 1957, *7,* 305-315.

Hunt, D. P. Effects of nonlinear and discrete transformations of feedback information on human tracking performance. *Journal of Experimental Psychology,* 1964, *67,* 486-494.

Hurwitz, L. J., & Allison, R. S. Factors influencing performance in psychological testing of the aged. In A. T. Welford & J. E. Birren (Eds.), *Behavior, Aging, and the Nervous System.* Springfield, Illinois: Charles C Thomas, 1965. (Pp. 461-475.)

Hyman, R. Stimulus information as a determinant of reaction time. *Journal of*

Experimental Psychology, 1953, *45,* 188-196.

Inglis, J. Immediate memory, age, and brain function. In A. T. Welford & J. E. Birren (Eds.), *Behavior, Aging, and the Nervous System.* Springfield, Illinois: Charles C Thomas, 1965. (Pp. 88-113.)

Jacobs, J. Experiments in prehension. *Mind,* 1887, *12,* 75-79.

Jeeves, M. A., & Dixon, N. F. Hemisphere differences in response rates to visual stimuli. *Psychonomic Science,* 1970, *20,* 249-251.

John, I. D. Sequential effects in absolute judgments of loudness without feedback. In S. Kornblum (Ed.), *Attention and Performance IV.* New York: Academic Press, 1973. (Pp. 313-326.)

John, I. D. Information processing in absolute and comparative judgment tasks. In P. M. A. Rabbitt & S. Dornic (Eds.), *Attention and Performance V.* London: Academic Press, 1975. (Pp. 722-732.)

Jones, B. Role of central monitoring of efference in short-term memory for movements. *Journal of Experimental Psychology,* 1974, *102,* 37-43.

Jong, J. R. de. The effects of increasing skill on cycle time and its consequences for time standards. *Ergonomics,* 1957, *1,* 51-60.

Kabrisky, M. *A Proposed Model for Visual Information Processing in the Human Brain.* Urbana: University of Illinois Press, 1966.

Kabrisky, M., Tallman, O., Day, C. M., & Radoy, C. M. A theory of pattern perception based on human physiology. *Ergonomics,* 1970, *13,* 129-147.

Kalsbeek, J. W. H. On the measurement of deterioration in performance caused by distraction stress. *Ergonomics,* 1964, *7,* 187-195.

Kaplan, I. T., & Carvellas, T. Scanning for multiple targets. *Perceptual and Motor Skills,* 1965, *21,* 239-243.

Kaplan, I. T., Carvellas, T., & Metlay, W. Visual search and immediate memory. *Journal of Experimental Psychology,* 1966, *71,* 488-493.

Karlin, L. Effects of delay and mode of presentation of extra cues on pursuit-rotor performance. *Journal of Experimental Psychology,* 1965, *70,* 438-440.

Karlin, L., & Martz, M. J. Response probability and sensory-evoked potentials. In S. Kornblum (Ed.), *Attention and Performance IV.* New York: Academic Press, 1973. (Pp. 175-184.)

Katz, L. Effects of differential monetary gain and loss on sequential two-choice behavior. *Journal of Experimental Psychology,* 1964, *68,* 245-249.

Katz, M. S. Feedback and accuracy of target positioning in a homogeneous visual field. *American Journal of Psychology,* 1967, *80,* 405-410.

Kaufman, H., & Levy, R. M. A further test of Hick's law with unequally likely alternatives. *Perceptual and Motor Skills,* 1966, *22,* 967-970.

Kawwa, T. A survey of ethnic attitudes of some British secondary school pupils. *British Journal of Social and Clinical Psychology,* 1968, *7,* 161-168.

Kay, H. Learning of a serial task by different age groups. *Quarterly Journal of Experimental Psychology,* 1951, *3,* 166-183.

Kay, H. The effects of position in a display upon problem solving. *Quarterly Journal of Experimental Psychology,* 1954, *6,* 155-169.

Kay, H. Some experiments on adult learning. In *Old Age in the Modern World:* Report of the 3rd Congress of the International Association of Gerontology, London, 1954. Edinburgh: Livingstone, 1955. (Pp. 259-267.)

Keele, S. W. Movement control in skilled motor performance. *Psychological Bulletin*, 1968, *70*, 387-403.

Keele, S. W. Repetition effect: A memory-dependent process. *Journal of Experimental Psychology*, 1969, *80*, 243-248.

Keele, S. W., & Ells, J. G. Memory characteristics of kinesthetic information. *Journal of Motor Behavior*, 1972, *4*, 127-134.

Keys, A., Brozek, J., Henschel, A., Mickelsen, O., & Taylor, H. L. *The Biology of Human Starvation*. Minneapolis: University of Minnesota Press, 1950.

Killingsworth, J. S. Private communication, 1972.

King, P. H. M. Task perception and interpersonal relations in industrial training: II. *Human Relations*, 1948, *1*, 373-412.

Kirby, N. H. Sequential effects in serial reaction time. *Journal of Experimental Psychology*, 1972, *96*, 32-36.

Kirby, N. H. Sequential effects in serial reaction time. Unpublished thesis, University of Adelaide, 1974.

Kirby, N. H. Serial effects in an eight choice serial reaction time task. *Acta Psychologica*, 1975, *39*, 205-216.

Kirchner, W. K. Age differences in short-term retention of rapidly changing information. *Journal of Experimental Psychology*, 1958, *55*, 352-358.

Klein, R. M., & Posner, M. I. Attention to visual and kinesthetic components of skills. *Brain Research*, 1974, *71*, 401-411.

Kleinsmith, L. J., & Kaplan, S. Paired-associate learning as a function of arousal and interpolated interval. *Journal of Experimental Psychology*, 1963, *65*, 190-193.

Kleinsmith, L. J., & Kaplan, S. Interaction of arousal and recall interval in nonsense syllable paired-associate learning. *Journal of Experimental Psychology*, 1964, *67*, 124-126.

Klemmer, E. T. Simple reaction time as a function of time uncertainty. *Journal of Experimental Psychology*, 1957, *54*, 195-200.

Knapp, B. *Skill in Sport: The Attainment of Proficiency*. London: Routledge and Kegan Paul, 1963.

Knight, A. A. Unpublished Thesis. University of Birmingham, 1967.

Laabs, G. J. Retention characteristics of different reproduction cues in motor short-term memory. *Journal of Experimental Psychology*, 1973, *100*, 168-177.

Laabs, G. J. The effect of interpolated motor activity on the short-term retention of movement distance and end-location. *Journal of Motor Behavior*, 1974, *6*, 279-288.

La Berge, D., & Tweedy, J. R. Presentation probability and choice time. *Journal of Experimental Psychology*, 1964, *68*, 477-481.

Lamb, J., & Kaufman, H. Information transmission with unequally likely alternatives. *Perceptual and Motor Skills*, 1965, *21*, 255-259.

Laming, D. R. J. A statistical test of a prediction from information theory in a card-sorting situation. *Quarterly Journal of Experimental Psychology*, 1962, *14*, 38-48.

Laming, D. R. J. A new interpretation of the relation between choice-reaction time and the number of equiprobable alternatives. *British Journal of Mathematical and Statistical Psychology*, 1966, *19*, 139-149.

Lappin, J. S., & Disch, K. The latency operating characteristic: I. Effects of stimulus probability on choice reaction time. *Journal of Experimental Psychology*, 1972a, *92*, 419–427.

Lappin, J. S., & Disch, K. The latency operating characteristic: II. Effects of visual stimulus intensity on choice reaction time. *Journal of Experimental Psychology*, 1972b, *93*, 367–372.

Laszlo, J. I. The performance of a simple motor task with kinesthetic sense loss. *Quarterly Journal of Experimental Psychology*, 1966, *18*, 1–8.

Lawson, E. A. Decisions concerning the rejected channel. *Quarterly Journal of Experimental Psychology*, 1966, *18*, 260–265.

Leonard, J. A. Advance information in sensorimotor skills. *Quarterly Journal of Experimental Psychology*, 1953, *5*, 141–149.

Leonard, J. A. Tactual choice reactions: I. *Quarterly Journal of Experimental Psychology*, 1959, *11*, 76–83.

Leonard, J. A., Newman, R. C., & Carpenter, A. On the handling of heavy bias in a self-paced task. *Quarterly Journal of Experimental Psychology*, 1966, *18*, 130–141.

Leuba, H. R. Measuring the size of an ergonomics problem. Paper to 3rd International Congress of Ergonomics, Birmingham, 1967.

Lewis, R. E. F. Consistency and car-driving skill. *British Journal of Industrial Medicine*, 1954, *13*, 131–141.

Lincoln, R. S. Learning and retaining a rate of movement with the aid of kinesthetic and verbal cues. *Journal of Experimental Psychology*, 1956, *51*, 199–204.

Lindley, R. H. Association value, familiarity, and pronunciability ratings as predictors of serial verbal learning. *Journal of Experimental Psychology*, 1963, *65*, 347–351.

Lindsley, D. B. Emotion. In S. S. Stevens (Ed.), *Handbook of Experimental Psychology*. New York: John Wiley & Sons; London: Chapman & Hall, 1951. (Pp. 473–516.)

Loeb, M., & Binford, J. R. Vigilance for auditory intensity changes as a function of preliminary feedback and confidence level. *Human Factors*, 1964, *6*, 445–458.

Lorge, I. The influence of regularly interpolated time intervals upon subsequent learning. *Teachers College Contributions to Education*, No. 438, 1930.

Loveless, N. E. Direction-of-motion stereotypes: A review. *Ergonomics*, 1962, *5*, 357–383.

McEwen, J. C. Working conditions with different types of disability. *Ergonomics*, 1973, *16*, 669–677.

McGrath, J. E. A conceptual formulation for research on stress. In J. E. McGrath (Ed.), *Social and Psychological Factors in Stress*. New York: Holt, Rinehart & Winston, 1970. (Pp. 10–21.)

McGuigan, F. J., & MacCaslin, E. F. Whole and part methods in learning a perceptual motor skill. *American Journal of Psychology*, 1955, *68*, 658–661.

Mackworth, J. F. The effect of true and false knowledge of results on the detectability of signals in a vigilance task. *Canadian Journal of Psychology*, 1964, *18*, 106–117.

Mackworth, J. F. Decision interval and signal detectability in a vigilance task. *Canadian Journal of Psychology*, 1965, *19*, 111–117.

Mackworth, J. F. *Vigilance and Habituation*. Harmondsworth: Penguin, 1969.

Mackworth, J. F. *Vigilance and Attention*. Harmondsworth: Penguin, 1970.

Mackworth, J. F., & Taylor, M. M. The *d'* measure of signal detectability in vigilance-like situations. *Canadian Journal of Psychology*, 1963, *17*, 302–325.

Mackworth, N. H. *Researches on the Measurement of Human Performance*. Medical Research Council Special Report Series No. 268. London: H.M.S.O., 1950.

McNicol, D. *A Primer of Signal Detection Theory*. London: George Allen & Unwin, 1972.

Macpherson, S. J., Dees, V., & Grindley, G. C. The effect of knowledge of results on learning and performance II. Some characteristics of very simple skills. *Quarterly Journal of Experimental Psychology*, 1948, *1*, 68–78.

Macrae, A. W., & Holding, D. H. Guided practice in direct and reversed serial tracking. *Ergonomics*, 1965, *8*, 487–492.

Macrae, A. W., & Holding, D. H. Transfer of training after guidance or practice. *Quarterly Journal of Experimental Psychology*, 1966, *18*, 327–333.

Marshall, P. H. Recognition and recall in short-term motor memory. *Journal of Experimental Psychology*, 1972, *95*, 147–153.

Marteniuk, R. G., & Roy, E. A. The codability of kinaesthetic location and distance information. *Acta Psychologica*, 1972, *36*, 471–479.

Marteniuk, R. G., Shields, K. W., & Campbell, S. Amplitude, position, timing, and velocity as cues in reproduction of movement. *Perceptual and Motor Skills*, 1972, *35*, 51–58.

Martin, J. G. Rhythmic (hierarchical) versus serial structure in speech and other behavior. *Psychological Review*, 1972, *79*, 487–509.

Martin, P. R., & Fernberger, S. W. Improvement in memory span. *American Journal of Psychology*, 1929, *41*, 91–94.

Megaw, E. D. Directional errors and their correction in a discrete tracking task. *Ergonomics*, 1972a, *15*, 633–643.

Megaw, E. D. Direction and extent uncertainty in step-input tracking. *Journal of Motor Behavior*, 1972b, *4*, 171–186.

Megaw, E. D. Possible modification to a rapid ongoing programmed manual response. *Brain Research*, 1974, *71*, 425–441.

Melton, A. W., & Irwin, J. McQ. The influence of degree of interpolated learning on retroactive inhibition and the overt transfer of specific responses. *American Journal of Psychology*, 1940, *53*, 173–203.

Merkel, J. Die zeitlichen Verhältnisse der Willensthätigkeit. *Philosophische Studien*, 1885, *2*, 73–127.

Michaels, R. M. Tension responses of drivers generated on urban streets. *Bulletin of the Highway Research Board*, Washington, 1960, No. 271, 29–44.

Michon, J. A. *Timing in Temporal Tracking*. Soesterberg: Institute for Perception RVO-TNO, 1967.

Michon, J. A. Programs and "programs" for sequential patterns in motor behavior. *Brain Research*, 1974, *71*, 413–424.

Miller, G. A. The magical number seven, plus or minus two: Some limits on our capacity for processing information. *Psychological Review*, 1956, *63*, 81–97.

Milner, B. Memory and the medial temporal regions of the brain. In K. H. Pribram & D. E. Broadbent (Eds.), *Biology of Memory*. New York: Academic Press, 1970. (Pp. 29–50.)

Mira, E. *Psychiatry in War*. London: Chapman & Hall, 1944.

Mitchell, M. J. H., & Vince, M. The direction of movement of machine controls. *Quarterly Journal of Experimental Psychology*, 1951, *3*, 24–35.

Moray, N. Attention in dichotic listening: Affective cues and the influence of instructions. *Quarterly Journal of Experimental Psychology*, 1959, *11*, 56–60.

Morin, R. E. Factors influencing rate and extent of learning in the presence of misinformative feedback. *Journal of Experimental Psychology*, 1955, *49*, 343–351.

Morrisett, L., & Hovland, C. I. A comparison of three varieties of training in human problem solving. *Journal of Experimental Psychology*, 1959, *58*, 52-55.

Morton, J. Interaction of information in word recognition. *Psychological Review*, 1969, *76*, 165-178.

Mowbray, G. H. Simultaneous vision and audition: The comprehension of prose passages with varying levels of difficulty. *Journal of Experimental Psychology*, 1953, *46*, 365-372.

Mowbray, G. H., & Rhoades, M. V. On the reduction of choice-reaction times with practice. *Quarterly Journal of Experimental Psychology*, 1959, *11*, 16-23.

Mowrer, O. H. Preparatory set (expectancy)—some methods of measurement. *Psychological Monographs*, 1940, *52*, No. 233.

Murdock, B. B. The immediate retention of unrelated words. *Journal of Experimental Psychology*, 1960, *60*, 222-234.

Murdock, B. B. A test of the "limited capacity" hypothesis. *Journal of Experimental Psychology*, 1965, *69*, 237-240.

Murray, D. J. Vocalization-at-presentation and immediate recall, with varying presentation-rates. *Quarterly Journal of Experimental Psychology*, 1965, *17*, 47-56.

Murray, D. J. Vocalization-at-presentation and immediate recall, with varying recall methods. *Quarterly Journal of Experimental Psychology*, 1966, *18*, 9-18.

Murrell, K. F. H. Data on human performance for engineering designers: Controls. *Engineering*, 1957, *184*, 308-310.

Murrell, K. F. H. *Ergonomics*. London: Chapman & Hall, 1965.

Naus, M. J. Memory search of categorized lists: A consideration of alternative self-termination search strategies. *Journal of Experimental Psychology*, 1974, *102*, 992-1000.

Naylor, J. C., & Briggs, G. E. Effects of task complexity and task organization on the relative efficiency of part and whole training methods. *Journal of Experimental Psychology*, 1963, *65*, 217-224.

Neisser, U. Decision-time without reaction-time: Experiments in visual scanning. *American Journal of Psychology*, 1963, *76*, 376-385.

Neisser, U., & Beller, H. K. Searching through word lists. *British Journal of Psychology*, 1965, *56*, 349-358.

Neisser, U., Novick, R., & Lazar, R. Searching for ten targets simultaneously. *Perceptual and Motor Skills*, 1963, *17*, 955-961.

Nettelbeck, T. The effects of shock-induced anxiety on noise in the visual system. *Perception*, 1972, *1*, 297-304.

Nettelbeck, T. An experimental investigation of some parameters affecting individual differences in perception. Unpublished Thesis. University of Adelaide, 1973a.

Nettelbeck, T. Individual differences in noise and associated perceptual indices of performance. *Perception*, 1973b, *2*, 11-21.

Neu, D. M. A critical review of the literature on "absolute pitch." *Psychological Bulletin*, 1947, *44*, 249-266.

Newell, K. M. Knowledge of results and motor learning. *Journal of Motor Behavior*, 1974, *6*, 235-244.

Nickerson, R. S. Response times with a memory-dependent decision task. *Journal of Experimental Psychology*, 1966, *72*, 761-769.

Nickerson, R. S. Categorization time with categories defined by disjunctions and conjunctions of stimulus attributes. *Journal of Experimental Psychology*, 1967, *73*, 211-219.

Nickerson, R. S., & Feehrer, C. E. Stimulus categorization and response time. *Perceptual and Motor Skills*, 1964, *18*, 785–793.

Nishioka, A., Akiba, N., & Yamahira, J. Experiments on the prolonged vigilance task (I). *Institute for Science of Labor, Tokyo, Reports*, No. 17, 1960. (Pp. 23–30.)

Norman, D. A. Learning and remembering: A tutorial preview. In S. Kornblum (Ed.), *Attention and Performance IV*. New York: Academic Press, 1973. (Pp. 345–362.)

Oldfield, R. C. Apparent fluctuations of a sensory threshold. *Quarterly Journal of Experimental Psychology*, 1955, 7, 101–115.

Oldfield, R. C., & Zangwill, O. L. The acquisition of verbal repetition habits. *British Journal of Psychology*, 1938, *29*, 12–26.

Oostlander, A. M., & de Swart, H. Search-discrimination time and the applicability of information theory. *Journal of Experimental Psychology*, 1966, *72*, 423–428.

Paillard, J., & Brouchon, M. A proprioceptive contribution to the spatial encoding of position cues for ballistic movements. *Brain Research*, 1974, *71*, 273–284.

Patrick, J. The effect of interpolated motor activities in short-term motor memory. *Journal of Motor Behavior*, 1971, *3*, 39–48.

Pepper, R. L., & Herman, L. M. Decay and interference effects in the short-term retention of a discrete motor act. *Journal of Experimental Psychology*, 1970, *83* (2), Part 2.

Peters, W., & Wenborne, A. A. The time pattern of voluntary movements. *British Journal of Psychology*, 1936, *26*, 388–406, and *27*, 60–73.

Pew, R. W. The speed-accuracy operating characteristic. *Acta Psychologica*, 1969, *30*, 16–26.

Pew, R. W. Levels of analysis in motor control. *Brain Research*, 1974, *71*, 393–400.

Pierce, J. R., & Karlin, J. E. Reading rates and the information rate of a human channel. *Bell System Technical Journal*, 1957, *36*, 497–516.

Pierson, W. R. Body size and speed. *Research Quarterly*, 1961, *32*, 197–200.

Pike, R. Response latency models for signal detection. *Psychological Review*, 1973, *80*, 53–68.

Pitz, G. F., & Downing, L. Optimal behavior in a decision-making task as a function of instructions and payoffs. *Journal of Experimental Psychology*, 1967, *73*, 549–555.

Pollack, I. The information of elementary auditory displays. *Journal of the Acoustical Society of America*, 1952, *24*, 745–749.

Pollack, I. The information of elementary auditory displays II. *Journal of the Acoustical Society of America*, 1953a, *25*, 765–769.

Pollack, I. Assimilation of sequentially encoded information. *American Journal of Psychology*, 1953b, *66*, 421–435.

Posner, M. I. Characteristics of visual and kinesthetic memory codes. *Journal of Experimental Psychology*, 1967, *75*, 103–107.

Posner, M. I. *Cognition: An Introduction*. Glenview, Illinois: Scott, Foresman & Co., 1973.

Posner, M. I., & Klein, R. M. On the functions of consciousness. In S. Kornblum (Ed.), *Attention and Performance IV*. New York: Academic Press, 1973. (Pp. 21–35.)

Posner, M. I., & Konick, A. F. Short-term retention of visual and kinesthetic information. *Organizational Behavior and Human Performance*, 1966, *1*, 71–86.

Postman, L., & Goggin, J. Whole versus part learning of serial lists as a function of meaningfulness and intralist similarity. *Journal of Experimental Psychology*, 1964, *68*, 140–150.

Poulton, E. C. On prediction in skilled movements. *Psychological Bulletin*, 1957, *54*, 467–478.

Rabbitt, P. M. A. Response-facilitation on repetition of a limb movement. *British Journal of Psychology*, 1965, *56*, 303–304.

Rabbitt, P. M. A. Times for transitions between hand and foot responses in a self-paced task. *Quarterly Journal of Experimental Psychology*, 1966, *18*, 334–339.

Rabbitt, P. M. A. Time to detect errors as a function of factors affecting choice-response time. *Acta Psychologica*, 1967, *27*, 131–142.

Rabbitt, P. M. A. Repetition effects and signal classification strategies in serial choice-response tasks. *Quarterly Journal of Experimental Psychology*, 1968, *20*, 232–240.

Rabbitt, P. M. A., & Vyas, S. M. An elementary preliminary taxonomy for some errors in laboratory choice RT tasks. *Acta Psychologica*, 1970, *33*, 56–76.

Rabbitt, P. M. A., & Vyas, S. M. What is repeated in the "repetition effect"? In S. Kornblum (Ed.), *Attention and Performance IV*. New York: Academic Press, 1973. (Pp. 327–342.)

Rapoport, A. A study of disjunctive reaction times. *Behavioural Science*, 1959, *4*, 299–315.

Reid, L. S., Henneman, R. H., & Long, E. R. An experimental analysis of set: The effect of categorical restriction. *American Journal of Psychology*, 1960, *73*, 568–572.

Remington, R. J. Analysis of sequential effects in choice reaction times. *Journal of Experimental Psychology*, 1969, *82*, 250–257.

Remington, R. J. Analysis of sequential effects for a four-choice reaction time experiment. *Journal of Psychology*, 1971, *77*, 17–27.

Requin, J. Some data on neurophysiological processes involved in the preparatory motor activity to reaction time performance. *Acta Psychologica*, 1969, *30*, 358–367.

Reynolds, B. The effect of learning on the predictability of psychomotor performance. *Journal of Experimental Psychology*, 1952, *44*, 189–198.

Reynolds, B., & Adams, J. A. Motor performance as a function of click reinforcement. *Journal of Experimental Psychology*, 1953, *45*, 315–320.

Robinson, G., & Loess, H. Short-term retention of individual paired associates as a function of conceptual category. *Journal of Experimental Psychology*, 1967, *75*, 133–135.

Rosenquist, H. S. The visual response component of rotary pursuit tracking. *Perceptual and Motor Skills*, 1965, *21*, 555–560.

Rowe, R. S., & Ivinskis, A. Melodic interval discrimination and the influence of training. *Australian Journal of Psychology*, 1972, *24*, 187–192.

Rubin, G., Trebra, P. von, & Smith, K. U. Dimensional analysis of motion: 3. Complexity of movement pattern. *Journal of Applied Psychology*, 1952, *36*, 272–276.

Russell, W. R. *Brain Memory Learning*. London: Oxford University Press, 1959.

Sadler, T. G., & Mefferd, R. B. Fluctuations of perceptual organization and orientation: Stochastic (random) or steady state (satiation)? *Perceptual and Motor Skills*, 1970, *31*, 739–749.

Saldanha, E. L. An investigation into the effects of prolonged and exacting visual work. *M.R.C. Applied Psychology Research Unit Report* No. 243, 1955.

Saldanha, E. L. Alternating an exacting visual task with either rest or similar work. *M.R.C. Applied Psychology Research Unit Report* No. 289, 1957.

Sanders, A. F. Rehearsal and recall in immediate memory. *Ergonomics,* 1961, *4,* 25-34.

Schvaneveldt, R. W., & Chase, W. G. Sequential effects in choice reaction time. *Journal of Experimental Psychology,* 1969, *80,* 1-8.

Schmidt, R. A., & White, J. L. Evidence for an error detection mechanism in motor skills: A test of Adams' closed-loop theory. *Journal of Motor Behavior,* 1972, *4,* 143-153.

Schwab, R. S. Motivation in measurements of fatigue. In W. F. Floyd & A. T. Welford (Eds.), *Symposium on Fatigue.* London: H. K. Lewis & Co. for the Ergonomics Research Society, 1953. (Pp. 143-148.)

Seibel, R. Discrimination reaction time for a 1,023-alternative task. *Journal of Experimental Psychology,* 1963, *66,* 215-226.

Seibel, R., Christ, R. E., & Teichner, W. H. Short-term memory under work-load stress. *Journal of Experimental Psychology,* 1965, *70,* 154-162.

Sekuler, R. W., & Abrams, M. Visual sameness: A choice time analysis of pattern recognition processes. *Journal of Experimental Psychology,* 1968, *77,* 232-238.

Sells, S. B. On the nature of stress. In J. E. McGrath (Ed.), *Social and Psychological Factors in Stress.* New York: Holt, Rinehart & Winston, 1970. (Pp. 134-139.)

Seward, J. P. The structure of functional autonomy. *American Psychologist,* 1963, *18,* 703-710.

Seymour, W. D. *Industrial Training for Manual Operations.* London: Pitman, 1954a.

Seymour, W. D. Experiments on the acquisition of industrial skills. *Occupational Psychology,* 1954b, *28,* 77-89; Part 2. Ibid., 1955, *29,* 82-98; Part 3. Ibid., 1956, *30,* 94-104; Part 4. Assembly tasks. Ibid., 1959, *33,* 18-35.

Shaffer, L. H. Latency mechanisms in transcription. In S. Kornblum (Ed.), *Attention and Performance IV.* New York: Academic Press, 1973. (Pp. 435-446.)

Shaffer, L. H., & Hardwick, J. Typing performance as a function of text. *Quarterly Journal of Experimental Psychology,* 1968, *20,* 360-369.

Shannon, C. E., & Weaver, W. *The Mathematical Theory of Communication.* Urbana, Illinois: University of Illinois Press, 1949.

Shelly, M. W. Learning with reduced feedback information. *Journal of Experimental Psychology,* 1961, *62,* 209-222.

Sherif, M., Taub, D., & Hovland, C. I. Assimilation and contrast effects of anchoring stimuli on judgments. *Journal of Experimental Psychology,* 1958, *55,* 150-155.

Sherwood, J. J. A relation between arousal and performance. *American Journal of Psychology,* 1965, *78,* 461-465.

Simon, H. A. An information-processing explanation of some perceptual phenomena. *British Journal of Psychology,* 1967, *58,* 1-12.

Simon, J. R., Hinrichs, J. V., & Craft, J. L. Auditory S-R compatibility: Reaction time as a function of ear-hand correspondence and ear-response-location correspondence. *Journal of Experimental Psychology,* 1970, *86,* 97-102.

Simon, J. R., & Simon, B. P. Duration of movements in a dial setting task as a function of the precision of manipulation. *Journal of Applied Psychology,* 1959, *43,* 389-394.

Simonson, E., & Brozek, J. Flicker-fusion frequency. Background and applications. *Physiological Reviews,* 1952, *32,* 349-378.

Singleton, W. T. Deterioration of performance on a short-term perceptual-motor task. In W. F. Floyd & A. T. Welford (Eds.), *Symposium on Fatigue.* London:

H. K. Lewis & Co. for the Ergonomics Research Society, 1953. (Pp. 163–172.)

Singleton, W. T. An experimental investigation of sewing-machine skill. *British Journal of Psychology*, 1957, *48*, 127–132.

Singleton, W. T., Easterby, R. S., & Whitfield, D. J. (Eds.) The human operator in complex systems. *Ergonomics*, 1967, *10*, 99–292.

Slack, C. W. Learning in simple one-dimensional tracking. *American Journal of Psychology*, 1953, *66*, 33–44.

Slamecka, N. J. Recall and recognition in list-discrimination tasks as a function of the number of alternatives. *Journal of Experimental Psychology*, 1967, *74*, 187–192.

Smith, G. A. Studies in compatibility and a new model of choice reaction time. In S. Dornic (Ed.), *Attention and Performance VI*. To be published, 1976.

Smith, K. U. *Delayed Sensory Feedback and Behavior*. Philadelphia: Saunders, 1962.

Smith, K. U., & Smith, W. M. *Perception and Motion*. Philadelphia: Saunders, 1962.

Solomons, L. M. A new explanation of Weber's law. *Psychological Review*, 1900, *7*, 234–240.

Spencer, J. Estimating averages. *Ergonomics*, 1961, *4*, 317–328.

Spencer, J. A further study of estimating averages. *Ergonomics*, 1963, *6*, 255–265.

Sperling, G. The information available in brief visual presentations. *Psychological Monographs*, 1960, *74*, No. 11.

Spielberger, C. D., & Denny, J. P. Visual recognition thresholds as a function of verbal ability and word frequency. *Journal of Experimental Psychology*, 1963, *65*, 597–602.

Spooner, A., & Kellogg, W. N. The backward conditioning curve. *American Journal of Psychology*, 1947, *60*, 321–334.

Stauffacher, J. C. The effect of induced muscular tension upon various phases of the learning process. *Journal of Experimental Psychology*, 1937, *21*, 26–46.

Stelmach, G. E., & Walsh, M. F. Response biasing as a function of duration and extent of positioning acts. *Journal of Experimental Psychology*, 1972, *92*, 354–359.

Sternberg, S. Memory scanning: Mental processes revealed by reaction-time experiments. *American Scientist*, 1969a, *57*, 421–457.

Sternberg, S. The discovery of processing stages: Extensions of Donders' method. *Acta Psychologica*, 1969b, *30*, 276–315.

Sternberg, S. Memory scanning: New findings and current controversies. *Quarterly Journal of Experimental Psychology*, 1975, *27*, 1–32.

Swets, J. A., & Sewall, S. T. Invariance of signal detectability over stages of practice and levels of motivation. *Journal of Experimental Psychology*, 1963, *66*, 120–126.

Swets, J. A., Tanner, W. P., & Birdsall, T. G. Decision processes in perception. *Psychological Review*, 1961, *68*, 301–340.

Symonds, Sir Charles. Disorders of memory. *Brain*, 1966, *89*, 625–644.

Szafran, J., & Welford, A. T. On the relation between transfer and difficulty of initial task. *Quarterly Journal of Experimental Psychology*, 1950, *2*, 88–94.

Tanner, W. P., & Swets, J. A. A decision-making theory of visual detection. *Psychological Review*, 1954, *61*, 401–409.

Taub, H. A., & Myers, J. L. Differential monetary gains in a two-choice situation. *Journal of Experimental Psychology*, 1961, *61*, 157–162.

Taylor, D. H. Drivers' galvanic skin response and the risk of accident. *Ergonomics*, 1964, *7*, 439–451.

Taylor, F. V., & Birmingham, H. P. Studies of tracking behavior. II. The acceleration pattern of quick manual corrective responses. *Journal of Experimental Psychology*, 1948, *38*, 783-795.

Taylor, F. V., & Garvey, W. D. The limitation of a "Procrustean" approach to the optimization of man-machine systems. *Ergonomics*, 1959, *2*, 187-194.

Taylor, J. A. A personality scale of manifest anxiety. *Journal of Abnormal and Social Psychology*, 1953, *48*, 285-290.

Teichner, W. H., & Krebs, M. J. Laws of visual choice reaction time. *Psychological Review*, 1974, *81*, 75-98.

Theios, J., Smith, P. G., Haviland, S. E., Traupmann, J., & Moy, M. C. Memory scanning as a serial self-terminating process. *Journal of Experimental Psychology*, 1973, *97*, 323-336.

Thierman, T. A signal detection approach to the study of set in tachistoscopic recognition. *Perceptual and Motor Skills*, 1968, *27*, 96-98.

Thomas, L. F. Perceptual organization in industrial inspectors. *Ergonomics*, 1962, *5*, 429-434.

Thorndike, E. L. *Human Learning*. New York: Appleton-Century, 1931.

Thorsheim, H. I., Houston, L., & Badger, C. Visual and kinesthetic components of pursuit-tracking performance. *Journal of Motor Behavior*, 1974, *6*, 199-203.

Thouless, R. H. Phenomenal regression to the "real" object. II. *British Journal of Psychology*, 1931, *22*, 1-30.

Thurstone, L. L. A law of comparative judgment. *Psychological Review*, 1927a, *34*, 273-286.

Thurstone, L. L. Psychophysical analysis. *American Journal of Psychology*, 1927b, *38*, 368-389.

Tolin, P. Effect of association value in a memory scan task. *Psychological Reports*, 1975, *37*, 3-6.

Tolin, P., & Delegans, G. M. The effect of stimulus complexity on retrieval of information from memory. *Memory and Cognition*, 1973, *1*, 380-382.

Training Made Easier: A Review of Four Recent Studies. D.S.I.R. Problems of Progress in Industry No. 6. London: H.M.S.O., 1960.

Trebra, P. von, & Smith, K. U. The dimensional analysis of motion: 4. Transfer effects and direction of movement. *Journal of Applied Psychology*, 1952, *36*, 348-353.

Treisman, A. M. Contextual cues in selective listening. *Quarterly Journal of Experimental Psychology*, 1960, *12*, 242-248.

Treisman, A. M. Verbal cues, language, and meaning in selective attention. *American Journal of Psychology*, 1964a, *77*, 206-219.

Treisman, A. M. The effect of irrelevant material on the efficiency of selective listening. *American Journal of Psychology*, 1964b, *77*, 533-546.

Treisman, A. M., & Geffen, G. Selective attention: Perception or response? *Quarterly Journal of Experimental Psychology*, 1967, *19*, 1-17.

Treisman, A. M., & Riley, J. G. A. Is selective attention selective perception or selective response? A further test. *Journal of Experimental Psychology*, 1969, *79*, 27-34.

Tresselt, M. E., & Volkmann, J. The production of uniform opinion by nonsocial stimulation. *Journal of Abnormal and Social Psychology*, 1942, *37*, 234-243.

Tsao, J. C. Studies in spaced and massed learning: 1. Time period and amount of practice. *Quarterly Journal of Experimental Psychology*, 1948, *1*, 29-36.

Ulehla, Z. J. Optimality of perceptual decision criteria. *Journal of Experimental Psychology*, 1966, *71*, 564-569.

Vernon, H. M. On the extent and effects of variety in repetitive work. *Industrial Fatigue Research Board Report* No. 26. London: H.M.S.O., 1924.

Verville, E., & Cameron, N. Age and sex differences in the perception of incomplete pictures by adults. *Journal of Genetic Psychology*, 1946, *68*, 149-157.

Vickers, D. Evidence for an accumulator model of psychophysical discrimination. *Ergonomics*, 1970, *13*, 37-58.

Vickers, D. A cyclic decision model of perceptual alternation. *Perception*, 1972, *1*, 31-48.

Vickers, D. Perceptual economy and the impression of visual depth. *Perception and Psychophysics*, 1971, *10*, 23-27.

Vickers, D., Nettelbeck, T., & Willson, R. J. Perceptual indices of performance: The measurement of "inspection time" and "noise" in the visual system. *Perception*, 1972, *1*, 263-295.

Vince, M. A. The intermittency of control movements and the psychological refractory period. *British Journal of Psychology*, 1948a, *38*, 149-157.

Vince, M. A. Corrective movements in a pursuit task. *Quarterly Journal of Experimental Psychology*, 1948b, *1*, 85-103.

Vince, M. A., & Welford, A. T. Time taken to change the speed of a response. *Nature*, 1967, *213*, 532-533.

Volkmann, A. W. Über den Einfluss der Übung auf das Erkennen räumlicher Distanzen. *Bericht Sächsische Akademie der Wissenschaften*, 1858, *10*, 38-69. Cited by Woodworth, 1938.

Vorro, J. R. Stroboscopic study of motion changes that accompany modifications and improvements in a throwing performance. *Research Quarterly*, 1973, *44*, 216-226.

Wachtel, P. L. Conceptions of broad and narrow attention. *Psychological Bulletin*, 1967, *68*, 417-429.

Walker, E. L., & Tarte, R. D. Memory storage as a function of arousal and time with homogenous and heterogenous lists. *Journal of Verbal Learning and Verbal Behaviour*, 1963, *2*, 113-119.

Wallace, J. G. Some studies of perception in relation to age. *British Journal of Psychology*, 1956, *47*, 283-297.

Wallace, R. J. S-R compatibility and the idea of a response code. *Journal of Experimental Psychology*, 1971, *88*, 354-360.

Ward, N. Speed as a function of distance: An analysis of road-cycling performances. *British Journal of Psychology*, 1950, *40*, 212-216.

Waugh, N. C. Serial position and the memory span. *American Journal of Psychology*, 1960, *73*, 68-79.

Waugh, N. C., & Norman, D. A. Primary memory. *Psychological Review*, 1965, *72*, 89-104.

Wehrkamp, R., & Smith, K. U. Dimensional analysis of motion: 2. Travel-distance effects. *Journal of Applied Psychology*, 1952, *36*, 201-206.

Welford, A. T. *Aging and Human Skill*. Oxford University Press for the Nuffield Foundation, 1958. Reprinted Westport, Connecticut: Greenwood Press, 1973.

Welford, A. T. *Ergonomics of Automation*. D.S.I.R. Problems of Progress in Industry No. 8. London: H.M.S.O., 1960a.

Welford, A. T. The measurement of sensory-motor performance: Survey and reappraisal of twelve years' progress. *Ergonomics*, 1960b, *3*, 189–230.

Welford, A. T. Experimental psychology in the study of ageing. *British Medical Bulletin*, 1964, *20*(1), 65–69.

Welford, A. T. Stress and achievement. *Australian Journal of Psychology*, 1965, *17*, 1–11.

Welford, A. T. Individual capacity and social demands: A new look at social psychology. In J. R. Lawrence (Ed.), *Operational Research and the Social Sciences*. London: Tavistock Publications, 1966a. (Pp. 531–542.)

Welford, A. T. The ergonomic approach to social behaviour. *Ergonomics*, 1966b, *9*, 357–369.

Welford, A. T. Single-channel operation in the brain. *Acta Psychologica*, 1967, *27*, 5–22.

Welford, A. T. *Fundamentals of Skill*. London: Methuen, 1968.

Welford, A. T. *Christianity—A Psychologist's Translation*. London: Hodder & Stoughton, 1971a.

Welford, A. T. What is the basis of choice reaction-time? *Ergonomics*, 1971b, *14*, 679–693.

Welford, A. T. Attention, strategy, and reaction time: A tentative metric. In S. Kornblum (Ed.), *Attention and Performance IV*. New York: Academic Press, 1973. (Pp. 37–53.)

Welford, A. T. Display layout, strategy, and reaction time: Tests of a model. In P. M. A. Rabbitt & S. Dornic (Eds.), *Attention and Performance V*. London: Academic Press, 1975. (Pp. 470–484.)

Welford, A. T., Brown, R. A., & Gabb, J. E. Two experiments on fatigue as affecting skilled performance in civilian air crew. *British Journal of Psychology*, 1950, *40*, 195–211.

Welford, N. T. An electronic digital recording machine—the SETAR. *Journal of Scientific Instruments*, 1952, *29*, 1–4.

West, L. J. Vision and kinesthesis in the acquisition of typewriting skill. *Journal of Applied Psychology*, 1967, *51*, 161–166.

White, R. W. Motivation reconsidered: The concept of competence. *Psychological Review*, 1959, *66*, 297–333.

Wickelgren, W. A. Size of rehearsal group and short-term memory. *Journal of Experimental Psychology*, 1964, *68*, 413–419.

Wickelgren, W. A. Short-term recognition memory for single letters and phonemic similarity of retroactive interference. *Quarterly Journal of Experimental Psychology*, 1966a, *18*, 55–62.

Wickelgren, W. A. Phonemic similarity and interference in short-term memory for single letters. *Journal of Experimental Psychology*, 1966b, *71*, 396–404.

Wickelgren, W. A. Rehearsal grouping and hierarchical organization of serial position cues in short-term memory. *Quarterly Journal of Experimental Psychology*, 1967, *19*, 97–102.

Wickelgren, W. A. Sparing of short-term memory in an amnesic patient: Implications for strength theory of memory. *Neuropsychologia*, 1968, *6*, 235–244.

Wilkinson, R. T. Artificial "signals" as an aid to an inspection task. *Ergonomics*, 1964, *7*, 63–72.

Wilkinson, R. T. Evoked response and reaction time. *Acta Psychologica*, 1967, *27*, 235–245.

Williams, A. C., & Briggs, G. E. On-target versus off-target information and the acquisition of tracking skill. *Journal of Experimental Psychology*, 1962, *64*, 519-525.

Williams, H. L., Beaver, W. S., Spence, M. T., & Rundell, O. H. Digital and kinesthetic memory with interpolated information processing. *Journal of Experimental Psychology*, 1969, *80*, 530-536.

Woodworth, R. S. The accuracy of voluntary movement. *Psychological Review Monograph Supplements*, 1899, *3*, No. 3.

Woodworth, R. S. *Experimental Psychology*. New York: Henry Holt & Co., 1938. 3rd Edition with H. Schlosberg. New York: Holt, 1954.

Woodworth, R. S. *Dynamics of Behavior*. New York: Henry Holt & Co.; London: Methuen, 1958.

Wright, J. M. von. *An Experimental Study of Human Serial Learning*. Societas Scientiarum Fennica. Commentationes Humanarum Litterarum, 1957a, *23*, No. 1.

Wright, J. M. von. A note on the role of "guidance" in learning. *British Journal of Psychology*, 1957b, *48*, 133-137.

Wyatt, S., & Langdon, J. N. Inspection processes in industry. *M.R.C. Industrial Health Research Board Report No. 63*. London: H.M.S.O., 1932.

Yerkes, R. M., & Dodson, J. D. The relation of strength of stimulus to rapidity of habit formation. *Journal of Comparative Neurology and Psychology*, 1908, *18*, 459-482.

Zangwill, O. L. An investigation of the relationship between the processes of reproducing and recognizing simple figures, with special reference to Koffka's trace theory. *British Journal of Psychology*, 1937, *27*, 250-276.

Zangwill, O. L. Some relations between reproducing and recognizing prose material. *British Journal of Psychology*, 1939, *29*, 370-382.

Zubek, J. P. Effects of prolonged sensory and perceptual deprivation. *British Medical Bulletin*, 1964, *20*(1), 38-42.

Author Index

Dale, H. C. A., 103, 114
Dardano, J. F., 146
Darrow, C. W., 135
Davies, D. R., 134, 146
Davis, D. R., 109, 142, 147
Davis, R., 72, 114
Davis, S. W., 141
Dees, V., 10
Delegans, G. M., 111
Delin, P. S., 115
Dember, W. N., 127
Denny, J. P., 112
Dijkstra, S., 103, 106
Disch, K., 68
Dixon, N. F., 71
Dodson, J. D., 135
Donders, F. C., 4
Downing, L., 22
Downs, S. M., 9, 109
Duncan, C. P., 116

Eagle, M. N., 115
Earhard, B., 52
Earl, R. W., 127
Eason, R. G., 146
Eccles, J. C., 119, 136
Ecob, J. R., 111
Edwards, W., 22
Egeth, H., 37
Ells, J. G., 85
El-Temamy, M. A. A., 86
Erdmann, R. L., 52
Eriksen, C. W., 53
Eysenck, H. J., 137

Feehrer, C. E., 39
Fernberger, S. W., 102
Filbey, R. A., 71
Fine, B. J., 137
Fitts, P. M., 59, 69, 72, 84
Foster, H., 39
Fraser, D. C., 160
Freeman, G. L., 134
Freud, S., 43
Furneaux, W. D., 138

Gabb, J. E., 106, 143
Garner, W. R., 53
Garvey, W. D., 75
Gates, A. I., 8, 105
Gazzaniga, M. S., 71
Geffen, G., 38
Gerhard, D. J., 96
Gibbs, C. B., 10–11, 87, 128
Gibson, J. J., 48–49, 50–51, 53
Gilbert, R. W., 118
Gilinsky, A. S., 50
Glanzer, M., 47
Glickman, S. E., 7
Goetz, E. T., 118
Goggin, J., 114
Goldman-Eisler, F., 89
Goldstein, M., 121
Goodeve, P. J., 82–83
Gordon, I. E., 4, 39
Gottwald, R. L., 53
Grandjean, E., 141
Gray, J. A., 8
Green, D. M., 18
Gregory, M., 146
Gregory, R. L., 14, 50
Griew, S., 71
Grindley, G. C., 10

Hale, D. J., 77
Hamilton, P., 145
Harcourt, R. A. F., 154
Hardwick, J., 93
Harter, N., 6
Haythorn, W. W., 160
Hebb, D. O., 7, 131, 136
Hebron, M. E., 127
Henderson, A., 89
Henri, V., 101
Herman, L. M., 5, 103
Hick, W. E., 56–62, 86
Hilgendorf, L., 38
Hochberg, J., 46
Hockey, G. R. J., 145
Hodge, M. H., 24
Holding, D. H., 108–109, 118
Hovland, C. I., 116
Howard, T. C., 22
Howell, W. C., 59

Hubel, D. H., 41
Hulbert, S. F., 11
Hunt, D. P., 118
Hurwitz, L. J., 113
Hyman, R., 58–60, 65, 77

Inglis, J., 104
Irwin, J. McQ., 114
Ivinskis, A., 27

Jacobs, J., 102
Jeeves, M. A., 71
Joffe, R., 142
John, I. D., 26–27
Jones, B., 118
Jong, J. R. de, 122

Kabrisky, M., 41, 51
Kalsbeek, J. W. H., 95
Kantowitz, B. H., 5
Kaplan, I. T., 39
Kaplan, S., 134
Karlin, J. E., 73
Karlin, L., 76, 119
Katz, L., 22
Katz, M. S., 118
Kaufman, H., 72
Kawwa, T., 153
Kay, H., 71, 106, 121
Keele, S. W., 77, 84–85
Kellogg, W. N., 120
Keys, A., 43
Killingsworth, J. S., 138
King, P. H. M., 100
Kirby, N. H., 77–78
Kirchner, W. K., 104
Klein, R. M., 5, 95
Kleinsmith, L. J., 134
Klemmer, E. T., 76
Knapp, B., 104–105
Knight, A. A., 72
Konick, A. F., 103, 106
Krebs, M. J., 72
Kreidler, D. L., 59

Laabs, G. J., 85, 103
La Berge, D., 111
Lamb, J., 72
Laming, D. R. J., 22, 62
Langdon, J. N., 146
Lappin, J. S., 68
Laszlo, J. I., 11
Lawson, E. A., 38
Leonard, J. A., 4, 69–70, 77, 94, 101
Leuba, H. R., 154
Levy, R. M., 72
Lewis, R. E. F., 122
Lincoln, R. S., 119
Lindley, R. H., 114
Lindsley, D. B., 135
Loeb, M., 146
Loess, H., 114
Lorge, I., 105
Loveless, N. E., 74
Luce, R. D., 62

McAlister, E., 46
MacCaslin, E. F., 104
McEwen, J. C., 139, 160
McGrath, J. E., 126, 128
McGuigan, F. J., 104
Mackworth, J. F., 145–146
Mackworth, N. H., 146
McNicol, D., 18
Macpherson, S. J., 10
Macrae, A. W., 108–109
Mahneke, A., 141, 145
Marshall, P. H., 118
Marteniuk, R. G., 85
Martin, J. G., 96
Martin, P. R., 102
Martz, M. J., 76
Mefferd, R. B., 32
Megaw, E. D., 11
Melton, A. W., 114
Merkel, J., 57, 72
Michaels, R. M., 11
Michon, J. A., 93, 96
Miller, G. A., 23–24, 102
Milner, B., 9
Mira, E., 135
Mitchell, M. J. H., 74–75
Moray, N., 38

Subject Index

Delinquency, 139
Dichotic listening, 8, 37–38
Discrimination, 16–21, 25, 32, 39, 52,
    62, 81, 135, 137
    of memory traces, 114
    See also Reaction times
Disorganization of performance,
    135,143
Displacement activities, 129
Diurnal rhythm, 137
Dominant details, 116
Driving, 4, 11, 66, 91, 122, 137, 147

Economy of performance, 2, 102, 147
Education, 14, 138
Effector mechanism, 3–4, 10, 12,
    82–83, 86–87, 92, 94, 96, 99
Efficiency. *See* Skill
Emotion. *See* Arousal
Ergonomics, 12
Errors
    arousal and, 133–34
    of choice, 67–69
    correction of, 10, 87–88, 147
    of decision, 20, 33, 81, 133–34
    ingraining of, 106–109, 120
    of memory, 102, 112
    and overloading, 89, 142–43
    of perception, 47, 152
    and reaction time, 58–59, 67–69, 77
    of timing, 96
Examination performance, 138
Exercise, 13
Expectancy, 12, 37, 42, 75, 78, 146, 147
Experience
    effects of, 12–14, 22, 37, 80, 99, 123,
        151
    predominance of initial, 14, 106
Extraversion-Introversion, 137–38, 160

Familiarity, effects of, 37, 42, 51–53,
    72, 94, 111, 114
Fatigue, 105–106, 140–45, 146–47
    mental, 141–45
    physical, 140–41
    and skill, 124, 147
    theories of, 144–45

Fear, 135, 152
Feedback, 9–10, 12, 80, 92–93
    and correction of errors, 87–89
    delayed, 5
    individual differences, 139
    and learning, 101, 118–20, 122
    and motivation, 127–28
    social, 150, 155–59
Flexibility of performance, 2, 10, 83,
    93, 116, 120, 124, 156
Foreperiod, 75–76
Fourier analysis, 41, 51
Friendship, 157–58
Frustration, 128, 140

Games, 11, 12, 80, 120
Gestalt school, 36

Habituation, 41, 130
Hick's law, 56–61, 68, 90
Hostility, 153, 157–59, 160
Human engineering, 12

Iconic storage, 8, 34
Identification, 41, 42, 44, 56, 59, 70,
    93, 112
Incentives, 22, 119, 127–28, 135–36
Individual differences, 13, 34, 51, 75,
    137–40
Industrial operations
    control and monitoring, 54, 75, 91,
        145
    and fatigue, 142
    high-speed, 97
    inspection, 53, 145
    and monotony, 146
    repetitive, 95, 124
    sensory discrimination, 28–29
    skilled, 1, 10, 12, 150
    training for, 109, 119, 121
Industrial organization, 124, 154–56
Information (theory), 36, 56–61, 65,
    72–73, 86, 89, 110, 130, 154, 156
Inspection (time), 29, 32–34, 64–67, 71,
    137–38
Intellectual capacity, 93

Intelligence, 75
Invariance in perception, 48, 50–52
Inverted-U hypothesis, 131–32, 138

Job satisfaction, 139, 156
Judgments, absolute, 23–28
    comparative, 28–34

Kinesthesis, 95, 121
Knitting, 91
Knowledge of results, 10, 118–19, 121,
    128, 146

Leadership, 154–56
Learning
    and arousal, 134
    and comprehension, 100–101, 104
    cumulative, 14, 99, 106
    difficult-easy transfer, 117–18
    "discovery," 109
    and feedback, 101, 118–20, 122
    guided, 108–109, 119
    by parts, 104
    and skill, 2
    stages of, 100, 120
Loading, 97, 104, 132, 140, 151–52,
    154–56
Loneliness, 157–59

Maturation, 13–14
Memory
    associations, 114–15
    economy in, 102
    effects of recall, 109
    errors of, 102, 112
    long-term, 4, 7, 9, 12, 92, 103,
        105–110, 112–15, 119, 134, 152
    and mental load, 97
    motor, 103
    retrieval, 89, 110–15. See also Recall,
        Recognition
    short-term, 4, 7–8, 22, 54, 92,
        101–105, 134, 143–44, 152
    traces, 7, 9, 100, 104, 110, 119–20,
        134, 136–37, 144

Mimic diagrams, 75
Monitoring, 88–89, 91–92, 95, 101, 147
Monotony, 11, 131, 137, 145–47, 160
Motivation, 10, 11, 43, 127–30, 140, 146
    hierarchical, 129, 139
    individual differences, 137–40
    optima, 10, 126, 130
Motor programming, 80–98, 147
Movement
    ballistic. See Action
    coordination of, 12, 94
    retention of, 103
    sequences, 91–93
    time, 60–61, 82–86
    velocity, 86, 116
Music, 6, 12, 80, 93, 96

Neuroticism. See Stability-Instability
Noise, random neural, 18–28, 32–34, 43,
    52, 59, 105, 132, 134, 136, 138, 144,
    146

Pacing. See Timing
Perception
    coding, 12, 36–54, 93, 99, 102, 106,
        147, 151
    constancy, 47, 49–52
    economy in, 36, 46, 49, 52, 54, 147
    fatigue effects, 141, 144
    frameworks in, 42, 53–54, 75
    gradients in, 48–51
    integration in, 45, 46–54
    mechanism, 4, 9–12, 40, 53, 78, 87–88,
        95, 106, 110, 118
    selection in, 36–45, 48
Perseveration. See Aftereffects
Personality, 34, 52, 137–38, 152, 154, 159
Population stereotypes, 74
Practice
    continuous (massed), 104
    effects of, 16, 29, 34, 45, 72, 78,
        93–96, 99, 118, 121–24, 147
    spaced, 105–106
Prediction, 80, 128, 130, 147, 155
Preparation, 76

Proprioception, 3
Psychiatric cases, 138–39, 159
Psychophysics, 16–34

Race relations, 152–53
Reaction time, 4–5, 80, 88, 142
  and attention, 63–64, 66
  and choice, 4, 53, 56–73, 81, 86, 110–11
  and compatibility. *See* Compatibility
  and discrimination, 29–34, 38, 53, 62,
    81, 111
  and errors, 31, 33, 58–59, 87
  and frequency, 58, 65, 78, 111
  sequential, 58, 75–78
  theoretical models, 56–69, 111, 113
Reading, 73, 93
Recall, 99–110, 114, 116, 134
Recognition, 114
Recruitment, 140, 144
Redundancy, 40, 89
Rehearsal, 105–106
Repetition effects, 76–78
Retardates, mental, 138–39
Reversible figures, 31
Rhythms, 96
Rigidity, 124

Scanning, 39, 45, 61, 110–11, 114
Schemata, 45, 52–53, 115
Sense organs, 3–4, 11–12, 40–41
Sequencing. *See* Timing
Serial processing, 44–45, 61–67
Signal detection theory, 18–27, 29
  and arousal, 132–33, 146
  β, 19–20, 22–23, 28, 145–46, 157
  cutoff, 19, 21, 25, 132–33, 136, 146
  optimum, 22, 132–33
  d', 19, 22–23, 28, 68, 145–46
  types of error, 20, 133
Signal-to-noise ratio. *See* Noise
Simultaneous processing, 44–45, 61–62,
  89
Simultaneous translators, 89
Single-channel hypothesis, 5–6, 11, 45,
  53, 76, 82, 87–92

Skill
  acquisition of. *See* Learning; Practice;
    Training
  definition of, 1–2
  efficiency, 2, 13, 66, 121, 124, 155
  fatigue and, 124, 147
  industrial. *See* Industrial operations;
    Industrial organization
  intellectual, 13, 93
  motivation, 127
  social, 13, 150–61
  stress effects on, 135, 147
  transfer of, 123
  types of, 12–14
Slips of the tongue, 43
Social
  interaction, 12, 130, 139, 150–61
  norms, 129, 153, 160
  stimulation, 157, 159–61
Spatial transposition, 71
Speed
  and accuracy, 58–59, 68, 81, 117, 142
  of continuous performance, 88
  and fatigue, 141–42, 144, 154
  of speaking, 89, 154
Sports. *See* Athletics; Games
Spread of effect, 68, 96–97, 102, 112,
  140, 144
Stability-Instability, 137–38
Stimulus–response theory, 5, 10, 80, 99
Storage. *See* Memory
Strategy, 2, 66–67, 71–72, 78, 81, 97, 102,
  111, 116
Stress
  conditions of, 126, 147, 152
  and difficulty, 135–36
  effects of, 11, 34, 75, 97, 128, 131–36
  individual differences, 136–40
Sublimation, 129
Symbolic recoding, 71
Systems, 2, 12, 150

Timing, 11, 95–97, 99, 105, 122, 142–43,
  147, 154
Threat, 128
Threshold, sensory, 17–18
Tracking, 4, 6, 75, 80, 86–88, 96, 108,
  116, 118–19, 122

Training
    effects of, 13–14, 16, 27, 29, 32, 34, 67, 75, 108, 126
    and flexibility, 116, 120
    length of session, 104
    methods, 51, 109
    pretraining, 100–101
    See also Learning
Translation mechanism, 4–6, 9–12, 53, 69–72, 78, 83, 86–88, 93–94, 96, 99, 101, 106, 110, 118
Typewriting, 6, 93, 107

Units of performance, 2, 6, 80–81, 93, 143, 147

Values, 129, 153, 160
Vigilance, 145–47, 160

Weber fraction, 17, 84

Yerkes-Dodson law, 135–36